Compulsive Eating:

A guide to end emotional eating, satisfy your hunger and form new habits. Discover how to stop binge disorder and the tips to never overeat again.

© Copyright 2019 - All rights reserved.

Table Of Contents

Introduction

It may seem complicated when you consider the various limits we have and how they fluctuate based on internal and external circumstances. The reality though, is that you'll figure yours out fairly easily once you start really paying attention.

It's simple—each time you feel regret, you've just discovered the location of another limit. You'll know that this time was an example of "too far" or "didn't work," so you can make an educated guess for doing better next time. Eventually, you'll have your limits fairly well mapped out and won't have to give them much ongoing thought. As you develop stronger habits for sticking with what works, you'll have more and more energy available for simply enjoying and appreciating your life. The longer you keep at this, the better you'll feel. Since you'll be approaching your life and eating patterns in a way that takes the best care of all parts of you, including your emotional brain, you won't be quietly seeking escape. It isn't that you'll never wobble; you almost certainly will, but it's likely to happen less often and less intensely over the years.

You'll enjoy clearer thinking, greater personal peace and integrity, a stronger, healthier body, and a much happier relationship with food. You'll probably lose your tolerance for feeling less than your physical and emotional best, which will strengthen your motivation even more.

You'll refine your practices over time, gradually honing an approach that works smoothly, effectively and with maximum satisfaction for you. You won't get it all figured out right away and you'll probably find that you need to fine-tune it periodically as your circumstances change, just as you do with other aspects of your life, but you'll get there. Someday, you may find that it no longer feels like a different thing that you're doing, but that it has simply become part of who you are and how you go through life.

Your personal process may go fairly smoothly, or not so much. It may gel quickly or seem to take forever to come together. Your weight may adjust to what you're hoping for or it may not. Regardless, you're likely to find that being on the road to getting better—even with potholes and detours—still feels better than being out of control.

I attended a seminar on nutrition some years ago, during which one of the speakers—while dispensing the usual guidelines for dieting—asserted, "Weight control is a lifelong project." While I did manage to contain myself, what I wanted to do was jump up and yell, "No! Life is a lifelong project!"

Life is about living. It's about growing and learning, loving and surviving grief, taking chances and learning to move forward through challenges, and about discovering how to be who you really are. It's about laughing and crying, singing and dancing. It's about playing, creating, sharing, and contributing. And at some point, it's about leaving, hopefully with a sense of having spent the time reasonably well. To look past all of that in favor of a narrow focus on weight is tragically to miss the point of making the most of our one, magnificent shot at this life. Perhaps the best thing about this new way of living with food is that you get to focus far more of your energy on living.

The Emotional Brain Revealed

Look no further than the nearest dog or cat to see most of what you need to know about the emotional brain. Like us, our pets have well-developed and powerful limbic systems but while our brains go on to develop much further, theirs do so only minimally. As a result, their behaviors and patterns nicely demonstrate how an emotional-brain-based life is lived.

We might like to think that our pets live on our terms, but the reality is that we have to work around them and have simply chosen the animals that require the least adjustment on our part. Dogs and cats are the most popular pets not just because they (usually) have such pleasing personalities, but because their natural behavioral tendencies are the easiest ones for us to live with. They are the most likely to be safe, enjoyable live-in companions for our families, eliminating their waste where we hope they will, and perhaps leaving most of our belongings unmolested.

The reason any number of other available animals have never caught on as pets is that we just can't adjust to the ways they tend to behave. If you doubt this, spend some time attempting to live with, say, a groundhog.

The point is that as much as we love them and as smart as we often think they are, our pets have only a limited, drive-based repertoire of responses. Their emotional brains are what give them the personalities we cherish, along with the following general characteristics:

If they really want to do something, you can't dissuade them unless you make the act immediately unpleasant for them or offer them an equally appealing alternative. Otherwise, you have to distract them until they forget about it, make it impossible for them to follow through, or just put up with them doing whatever it is.

If they don't want to do something, you can't change that, either. You have to find a way to trick or force them into doing it, or just give up and live without it happening at all.

They react strongly and without deliberation to perceived opportunities and threats, based only on what motivates them the most right in the moment (unless they've received considerable training for alternative behaviors). Their concept of the future is limited at best, so they have little capacity for planning and strategy. Their thinking would sound like, I want this! or, I need to get away! rather than, I can see how this is going to turn out and will choose accordingly.

They can only make connections between actions and results that occur nearly simultaneously. Most cause and effect relationships are beyond their comprehension because they have so little ability to understand how this moment relates to any other moment in time, be it five minutes ago or five minutes from now.

Now, consider the characteristics above as you think about the part of you that urgently goes after food in ways that repeatedly sabotage your health and peace of mind:

If you really want to eat something, you can't stop wanting it unless it is somehow made immediately unpleasant (like the snack you're obsessing over until you're able to squirt dishwashing liquid all over it) or you can identify an equally appealing alternative. Otherwise, you have to distract yourself and hope you can forget about it, make it impossible to obtain, or just give up and eat it so that at least the inner torment will stop.

If you don't want to do something (like exercising regularly), you can't make yourself want it even though you believe you should. You have to find a way to trick, bargain, or force yourself into it, or just give it up so that at least you're not fighting with yourself over it anymore.

You are triggered rapidly and intensely by your most tempting foods. You quickly lose your will to resist them or to have them in moderation. You'd like to be more deliberative in those moments—you truly would—but you just can't do it.

Your strongest feelings are based on how much you do or don't want to do something right now. Part of you knows you'll feel bad about this later, but that fails to outweigh the urgency you feel in the moment. You wonder how you could possibly not have learned the lesson yet after all the times it has gone this way before.

There you go—you've just met your emotional brain. As frustrated as you may presently feel with it, remember that this system works extremely well in settings of scarcity and hardship, which is all most of humanity has ever known until quite recently. It has a lot to do with our surviving and thriving enough to be here now.

In fact, we as a species have been so spectacularly successful that we've been able to remake our world, a world in which—ironically—the emotional brain is now tragically out of its element. In order to appreciate why that is so, it pays to understand some fundamentals about how this part of you works.

History of problem eating

Due to the limitation of space, it is not possible to discuss all eight of the eating disorder categories in detail, so I apologize in advance to any reader who may be concerned about one of the less common eating disorder conditions. But by including the diagnostic criteria, you will at least be able to recognize the symptoms and decide if you need to seek professional support by contacting your GP.

Problem eating is not a new phenomenon

Descriptions of difficult or unusual relationships with food can be found in ancient Persian, Chinese and Egyptian scrolls and hieroglyphics. Negative behaviours, such as purging and self-starvation are not new inventions; their incidence in populations varies in accordance with cultural and economic factors, among a host of other variables.

There are descriptions from the Hellenistic era that mention religious fasting leading to what we now term the illness of anorexia. It is important to note that although more evidence exists of females suffering from the various disorders throughout history, there is also clear evidence that males did not escape the clutches of these psychiatric afflictions.

Anorexia mirabilis

In the Middle Ages, a phenomenon known as anorexia mirabilis (miraculous absence of appetite) or 'holy anorexia' was in fashion among Catholic women as a means of demonstrating their purity and holiness. One of the most famous of these women was Saint Catherine of Siena, who lived in the 14th century and showed her devotion to Christ through celibacy and fasting.

Saint Catherine of Siena purged any food that she was made to eat by pushing twigs down her throat to make herself vomit. She died prematurely at the age of 33 as a result of starvation.

These sufferers believed that to survive without food showed that the spirit was more important than the body. By achieving this higher plane of spirituality, these deeply religious women were deemed to be closer to God. The women also pursued many other forms of penance and self-mortification to show evidence of their piety and humility, such as wearing hairshirts and performing self-flagellation.

Other notable historical figures believed to have suffered from anorexia are Saint Hedwig of Silesia (who, for the benefit of younger readers, was a duchess, not an owl), Mary Queen of Scots, Joan of Arc, Mary Tudor and Catherine of Aragon.

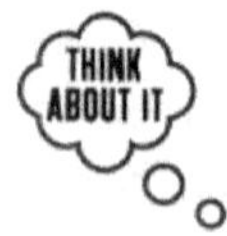

There is a distinct difference between the motivation of the sufferers of anorexia mirabilis and today's anorexia nervosa sufferers – the former used fasting as a means of communicating with Christ and the latter are troubled by body image and underlying emotional problems. However, the common thread between the two forms of anorexia is the sufferer's perception that they are exercising self-discipline, which in turn creates a sense of personal control.

Thwarting the survival instinct
This is because the self-imposed starvation causes the brain to malfunction and sufferers can no longer protect their own survival.

It is ironic that a quest intended to demonstrate self-discipline and autonomy leads to the sufferer's mind falling under the command of the eating disorder voice, with its insatiable desire for further weight loss, even if this ultimately results in death.

Early evidence of bulimia
Many people believe that bulimia first emerged in ancient Rome, with affluent Romans using a 'vomitorium' at banquets so that they could eat far more rich food than would otherwise be possible. In fact, a vomitorium was actually a passage used for easy egress from seats in an amphitheatre and not a place in which one could conveniently deposit one's lunch or dinner.

However, there is reliable evidence from the Middle Ages that wealthy people would vomit to enable themselves to eat more. Feasts and banquets in those days consisted of up to six courses. Courses would include vast quantities of goslings, rabbits, roe-deer, sturgeon, peacocks, swans, stuffed capons and wild boar and generous helpings of pastries and jellies of every description. One can appreciate the difficulty in accommodating such a bill of fare at one sitting, though clearly the obvious solution is to simply eat less.

Anorexia nervosa

Bulimia

Though the term had been around for a while, I believe it was Princess Diana's confession in the early 1990s that she suffered from bulimia that brought the condition to wider attention. This resulted in an avalanche of hidden sufferers coming out of the closet to seek help for this disabling illness.

Unlike anorexia, where the ravages of the disease are clearly visible, many people who suffer from bulimia can keep their problem hidden. This is because they are often able to maintain a normal weight and are therefore not readily identifiable. However, this does not mean that their psychological suffering or physical deterioration is any less acute than in those whose condition is visibly evident.

Binge eating disorder (BED)

There is scant historical evidence for binge eating disorder, also known as compulsive eating disorder. This is largely due to the fact that rather than being identified as a psychological or mental health problem, akin to addiction, in the past it was often erroneously simply attributed to greed.

Binge eating disorder is when a person repeatedly eats significantly more than what would be considered a normal amount of food within a limited time frame, and feels out of control while doing so.

Obesity

By and large, obesity, one of the potential consequences of binge eating disorder, appears to have not been overly prevalent in the past. Where it did occur, it was clearly the preserve of the aristocracy, as the poor working man and woman would not have been able to afford an excess of food.

Today, binge eating disorder is overwhelmingly the most common of the eating disorders for both males and females and is rising in many populations. Alarmingly, young children are falling prey to this disorder, as can be seen by the relatively recent rise of overweight and obese youngsters. Although a significant number of overweight people suffer from binge eating disorder, it is important to note that not all of them do.

Pica disorder

It is difficult to trace the history of the disorder with accuracy, since it was frequently seen as a symptom of other disorders. Further confusion arises with regard to diagnosis of pica disorder because of cultural norms differing within various societies. Thus, identical eating practices would be deemed normal within one population and pathological in another – for example, in parts of Africa it is common for pregnant woman to eat clay, but in the UK that would be considered unusual behaviour.

Geophagia

Geophagia is the ingestion of earthy substances such as clay, soil and chalk. The practice of clay ingestion is still popular in some cultures, where it is used as a form of medication, delivering various nutrients, such as phosphorus and sulphur, from the soil. In these circumstances it would not be diagnosed as pica disorder.

Pica

One of the earliest examples of pica is the Christian mystic Angela of Foligno, who in the 13th century managed to live to the age of 61 on very little food, supplemented with non-nutritious matter such as lice, scabs and the pus from the sores of the sick and dying. She was revered for these practices, which were seen as the antithesis of four of the seven cardinal sins: gluttony, greed, pride and lust.

Rumination disorder

Rumination refers to the involuntary regurgitation of food. Rumination is normal within certain animal species, such as giraffes and cows, and is known as chewing the cud, but it is considered pathological in humans and other animal populations such as gorillas where it has also been observed.

Well-documented accounts of rumination include a patient of an Italian anatomist in 1618 who suffered from what was then known as 'rumination syndrome'. Much later we have an account of a Mauritian physiologist, Charles Edouard Brown-Sequard, who in the mid-19th century conducted an experiment upon himself to discover the response of stomach acid to different food types. By swallowing food attached to sponges and strings, he inadvertently trained himself to regurgitate food without the need of mechanical assistance; rumination became habitual and no longer under voluntary control.

Rumination disorder is most prevalent in young children and people suffering from cognitive disabilities. A cognitively healthy adult who appears to have this issue may in fact have a physical problem. Rumination disorder can adversely affect normal functioning and has been linked with depression.

Avoidant/restrictive food intake disorder (ARFID)

This is a disorder in which the limitation of food intake is not connected with any concerns around weight and shape. This is usually only a phase, which children overcome naturally as they mature and does not require the need for medical intervention. However, a number of sufferers carry this disorder into their adult lives.

An ARFID sufferer might refuse to consume whole food groups such as vegetables and fruit. Alternatively, their choices may be based purely on the food's properties such as colour, texture, whether it is hot, cold, soft, chewy, crunchy, liquid or solid. Sufferers of ARFID will be very wary about trying out any new foods and will restrict themselves to what they regard as 'safe' foods. This anxiety will naturally impair the quality of their social life to varying degrees. When eating foods that they regard as 'unsafe' the sufferer may gag, retch or vomit, which will cause them enormous distress and reinforce their reticence in experimenting further with new types of food.

This extreme rigidity of food selection not only interferes with the sufferer's ability to socialize, but in extreme cases has proved fatal. In the pursuit of purity, many foods become proscribed, resulting in an inadequate diet, which can lead to malnutrition and death. Although on the surface this fixation on 'healthy' eating may not appear to have a mental health component, this is far from the case. It is often linked to the sufferer being phobic about ill health or having an overriding desire for control in order to increase self-esteem.

Bigorexia

Bigorexia is a form of muscle dysmorphia where the individual becomes obsessive-compulsive about building up their physique in a quest for perfection. This will not only involve excessive body-building exercises in the gym but will also have an impact on the sufferer's diet. It affects both men and women but is more common in men.

Sufferers of bigorexia will eat a low-fat, high protein diet combined with excessive amounts of food supplements. Their mental health suffers since their body perception becomes increasingly distorted; they work out even when injured or ill and some resort to steroid abuse. The intense workout regimes interfere with both their social and work life and some sufferers have become suicidal as the psychological toll of the dysmorphia becomes unbearable.

Body dysmorphia is when an individual becomes pathologically obsessed about the way they look and has a distorted perception of their own body. Some people may fixate on the shape of their nose or the size of a scar and exaggerate this perceived defect out of all proportion. Someone suffering from anorexia will see himself as fat when they are in fact emaciated. It is also known as the imagined ugliness disease since it bears no resemblance to objective reality.

Drunkorexia

Unlike bigorexia, drunkorexia predominantly affects females. Drunkorexia is linked to body image and weight and is an unhealthy attempt to reduce calorie intake while still being able to live the 'good life'. Sufferers skip meals so that their precious calorie intake can be reserved for alcohol, enabling them to be party animals.

The dangers of this form of behaviour are substantial in the long term, since it increases the risk of liver disease, dementia and diabetes. The short-term consequences are also significant in that excessive alcohol intake on an empty stomach increases intoxication levels and lowers inhibitions, which can lead to dangerous risk-taking behaviour. In the medium term, drunkorexia increases the chances of the sufferer becoming an alcoholic and/or developing a serious eating disorder.

Pregorexia

Pregorexia is the term used for pregnant women who have a terror of pregnancy-related weight gain. It should go without saying that this is an exclusively female problem! Sufferers of pregorexia mirror the behaviour of sufferers of anorexia in that they will restrict their calorie intake and exercise compulsively. Pregorexia may also be linked to a desire to exude an aura of control and purity as a reaction to the messiness of childbirth.

This behaviour can have very severe consequences for both the mother and the unborn child, not least pregnancy complications and premature childbirth. It is more prevalent in women who have suffered physical abuse, rape or other stressful events. A genetic predisposition has been identified, and the impact of chemical and hormonal imbalances have also been suggested as potential causes for the development of pregorexia.

How to Stop Emotional Eating

If you want to gain control over your life and stop emotional eating, you need to understand a few basic things. Firstly, it cannot be done in a single day just because you suddenly say you will stop eating that way. The problem is deep-rooted and will require some effort, but it's not impossible. Don't think of it as something too easy or too difficult. The first step is to identify the problem and then you can start dealing with it. It won't be a single step toward a healthier you but an entire process that this book will help you with. As you go step by step, you will slowly be able to stop eating unless you are truly hungry, and you will learn how to deal with your emotions in a healthier way.

Diagnosis of Emotional Eating

Many different health care providers or specialists help to evaluate and treat emotional eating. Over the years it has become a much more prevalent problem than it was a couple of decades ago. Emotional eating is a major contributing factor to obesity and excessive weight gain in people, and this has made professionals more aware of the need to deal with the problem. When you know that the problem is serious, it is best to consult a professional for help. You might need a consultation with a psychologist, help from a pediatrician, or monitoring of your eating. Sometimes just one doctor is enough to help you out, but for those who deal with a more severe problem like an associated eating disorder, multiple sources might be required.

The initial diagnosis of emotional eating is made after a proper physical examination and tests to check for any medical conditions or genetic factors. There are some standardized tests with questions for the patient to answer in order to assess the condition. The patient's mental health history is studied to check for eating disorders like pica or bulimia or any mental illnesses. All this together is used to determine whether the person suffers from emotional eating and the extent of it.

Identifying the Triggers of Emotional Eating

You need to start by identifying what triggers you to start eating when you're not even hungry. Think about the last few times you had sudden cravings or binged on food. Write these instances down on a list. Seeing it written down can be quite revealing and help you see the pattern of ignoring problems and eating to combat them. There can be many different reasons for emotional eating. To deal with your emotional eating, you must identify what triggers it. What kinds of situations, people, or feelings make you want to eat your comfort foods? Do you eat when you feel sad to drown your sorrows? Or do you eat when you want to celebrate an event? Does being around a particular person make you want to indulge in food to feel better? Everyone has different triggers, so don't shrug off a reason just because it seems normal to you. Some people are triggered when they are stress about work. You might be emotionally eating when you have to do something you didn't want to. You might compulsively eat every time you see food or pass by a food stall.

Maybe you eat every time you think of or hear about a particular food, or you feel obligated to eat just because you know it's lunch or dinnertime and can't seem to skip it even if you're not hungry. You might just keep eating whenever you're bored and have nothing to do. Some people eat more when they are stressed by the people around them, like relatives at a family gathering. All of these and many more could be triggers for your unhealthy emotional eating habits. Until you identify them, you cannot start to overcome the habit.

Ideally, everyone would eat only when they were hungry and only as much as their body really needed. We would all be able to stop eating as soon as our stomach was full and not hungry anymore; however, most of us eat a lot when affected by extrinsic factors like being part of a celebration or when dealing with stress. This is why you need to work on building a healthy relationship with food. Your attitude should be one of "eat to live" rather than "live to eat." Appreciating food is very different from being obsessed with it. An unhealthy relationship with food can be the root of many problems, both physically and emotionally. Identifying the triggers for your eating will make you more conscious of your actions in the future. You will become more aware of what you are doing every time you reach for food. Once you know your triggers, you have a better chance of dealing with them.

Understanding Your Reasons

Once you have written down all the triggers that lead to your emotional eating, try to understand why they affect you negatively. It may have seemed completely normal to eat that way in some situations, but when you compare your behavior to others', you will see the issue. For instance, if you go to a birthday party, it might seem compulsory for you to eat the cake, but your friend might say no. At that time, you probably thought it weird for them to refuse cake since it's a basic part of the occasion, but now that you question it, you realize it's just a conditioned habit and that you don't really have to eat it if you don't want to. The problem is that you never stopped to think about it and just ate the cake because it was there.

Start looking at the list of your triggers and question why each one affects you. Write down the answers beside the list. Don't write answers like "it's normal," but instead think about what makes you want to indulge in emotional eating in the moment of that particular trigger. Keep questioning yourself till you realize how you linked that particular situation to eating over the years.

Detach These Triggers from Food

After all the self-questioning, you know most of the reasons behind why these triggers prompt you to eat. The next step is to work toward disassociating food from these triggers. Try to understand how each link was established. At some point in the past, you started eating in response to a particular situation, and over time your body became conditioned to it. You need to identify what that situation was and accept that this link you established is not really normal and is very different from how other people react to the same situation. If you want to stop yourself from continuing the same self-destructive behavior, you first have to accept that it is not healthy and is incongruent with how others deal with situations.

Once you start accepting that it was wrong to link eating with those triggers, you will start understanding that it was all in your mind. In reality, the triggers don't have any relation to eating, and you shouldn't link them in that way. The triggers have to be separated from the eating since the two things are completely different issues. Eating should be linked only to physical hunger that has to be satisfied to provide the body with energy. The triggers that cause emotional eating are completely irrelevant to why you should eat.

For instance, think about how you associate food with celebrations. You will see that most celebrations in the past have had a lot of food involved. Thanksgiving tables are always filled with food, and everyone eats till they're stuffed and not just till their hunger is sated. As kids, we went to fast food places like McDonald's right after exams were over to celebrate with sodas and burgers. As adults, we treat ourselves to a fancy restaurant dinner when the paychecks come in. Celebrations have always been deemed incomplete without a lot of food to enjoy them with. This is why our brains are synced to associate food with celebrations every single time, but you need to realize that it's a very illogical way of thinking. Why do you need to eat excessive food to celebrate something good? It's not just the fact that you eat unhealthy food but also how much more you eat than necessary.

When there is something to celebrate, embrace the feeling of happiness it gives you. Process the emotion itself and don't do it with food. All that food will just counteract your positive feelings and make you punish yourself later when you gain extra weight. Everyone is always complaining about the holiday weight they gain after the festivities are over, but no one stops to think about why they eat so much in the first place. You can still eat some good meals during the holidays, but you don't have to indulge to the point where all your clothes stop fitting you. When you start to consciously think about this, you will slowly stop eating compulsively every time something good happens. Don't distract yourself with food but embrace the happy emotions by themselves.

Another example is dealing with cravings. Sudden cravings for food are one of the most common symptoms of emotional eating. Most of the time, these cravings are associated with junk food or any unhealthy food that gives you a momentary rush. When you have such cravings, you might think that it's a form of hunger and you absolutely have to satisfy it, but you need to start thinking about these cravings more and realize that they are linked only to your mind and not your body.

If you stop and ask yourself why you keep craving a particular food, you will understand better. Most of the time it's because you associate that food with something good that happened and eating it makes you feel better again. There are certain foods like pancakes or waffles that your mom might have treated you with when you were younger. As you grow older, eating these things imparts a sense of comfort and goodness in you again, but if you think about it, you felt good because of your mother and not the food. The food was just one way she showed you love, but it was not the root of it. If you want to feel better in a situation, think about her and not the food.

Deal with the Triggers

Emotional eating usually happens when you don't want to deal with a certain emotion or situation. In order to turn off this trigger, you need to first deal with it. Eating cannot act as a makeshift solution. If you don't deal with the problem and try to resolve it, it won't go away. Eating will just suppress your emotions and help you push the problem to the back of your mind. You might feel better and not think of it for a while, but it will continue to come forward until you actually resolve it. Because emotional eating is largely associated with stress, one of the most crucial aspects of this is stress management. As you read on, stress management will be dealt with in a more thorough manner to help you through it.

Another thing you need to deal with is straying from your diet. Most people with excessive weight gain try to go on diets to get healthier and lose weight. The first issue arises when they choose unhealthy fad diets that do more harm than good to the body. These diets are designed to make you fail, but even when you do find a healthy diet, you might occasionally slip up. It's okay if you eat something outside the confines of your diet once in a while; you don't need to punish yourself for it. Many people tend to stress out when this slipup happens, and then they go forward and binge-eat, which just makes it worse. Let go of the small stuff and focus on the big picture. Start saying no to food even if it is offered to you when you know you shouldn't be eating it. This simple no will help you avoid the stress of feeling guilty and the retaliation of overeating later.

Slowly but surely you will learn to deal with the triggers that make you eat emotionally. You need to address them if you want to solve the problem. Think about why you turn to food when a particular situation comes up and plan out how you will react and deal with it when it happens again. This will help you to turn away from emotional eating when you are stressed, lonely, or just feeling low about your body image.

The Role of Family and Society in Binge Eating

There are several misconceptions about what role the family of the person suffering from BED plays. More often than not the families are blamed for causing these disorders in their family member. But that's not true at all. It could be that the person suffering from binge eating has developed a personality that is not well equipped to handle difficult situations in life, the reason why they may resort to binge eating.

It's also possible that despite having a supportive family, the person might feel the need to keep his disorder a secret, and as a result does not receive any help from them. Eating disorders like binge eating can stem from a multitude of factors, and to say that families are responsible for causing their eating disorders would not be accurate.

In fact, being surrounded by your family is the best thing that can happen to an individual suffering from binge eating disorder.

It would also help if the person takes this time to reflect his or her relationship with the family to understand if it's any way responsible for their eating disorder.

The individual can start asking questions such as, *can I describe my relationship with my family as healthy? Does my family welcome unhealthy food? Was I a part of my family meals growing up? Was there an emphasis on superficial things like appearance, status, or external success in the family?* Finding answers to some or all of these questions may help a person understand the dynamics around food in the family, and how some of these factors have contributed towards their disorder.

An interesting exercise that most psychotherapists ask their patients to do is to create a living sculpture, or picture, that represents their family's relationship with food. Sometimes they may be asked to depict a family meal or picture themselves as a part of the meals.

This helps them identify the patterns around food that the individual may not be consciously aware of. These dynamics may not necessarily trigger eating disorders but helps the person get a valuable insight to understand their beliefs about food that may have been shaped by the family.

There are a lot of ways in which family can help a person with BED recover quickly.

Encourage them to get help

Treatment is vital when it comes to recovery of the person suffering from binge eating disorder. Getting help from a specialist might seem like an extreme idea to the individual, but the family can help him or her in understanding how it can positively impact them.

The individual may need a bit of convincing and this can only be done tactfully by close members of the family. It is important to remain supportive throughout the individual's recovery. It certainly is a slow road and it might take a lot of patience to get them to seek help, but it's definitely worth the trouble. You may suddenly have an AHA moment with them where they suddenly give in and agree to go to the doctor.

Refrain from making negative comments about them

This includes making any negative remarks about yourself too. Avoid talking about your body in a negative way. Do not make comments about people's eating habits, as binge eaters may be sensitive about such remarks even if they don't react in front of you.

You should be extra careful of saying anything that involves food or the shape of size of others or your own body. On the contrary, express empathy by using "I feel statements" such as, "I feel concerned about your eating habits. Help me understand what it's like to not be able to control your hunger."

Or if the person suffering from BED makes condescending remarks about his own self, say something like, "I love you the way you are, and I feel upset that you haven't been treating your body right."

Do not manipulate them into eating their meals on time

The hardest part about dealing with a binge eater is getting them to eat their meals on time. Honestly, you shouldn't even try to convince them. You need to understand that their appetites don't work the same as people without an eating disorder.

They only feel like eating when the cravings come calling and that's the only time they will consume whatever food you put in front of them on the table. Guilt-tripping them, bargaining or begging is only going to strain your relations with them.

For one, it won't shift their thinking, and they may start avoiding you because of your coaxing.

Encourage them to express their feelings

Listen to them when they feel out of control. Encourage them to open up to you about what they feel. If you suspect that they are going through some major trauma in their lives, take some time to get them to express their feelings.

Ask questions about their personal or professional life but be extremely tactful while doing so. You can't be forceful or demanding while doing so. Be gentle and be ready to listen whenever they feel like talking about it. People with BED often feel overwhelmed by their emotions as a result of which they tend to suppress their feelings a lot.

Just venting out to a family member about their issues can go a long way in helping them to come to terms with their problems. You can also encourage these individuals to express themselves through art, music or simply screaming for a bit.

If you are a close, get involved in their treatment

This could mean accompanying them during their regular consultations with the therapist or helping them watch their impulses. Stanford University conducted a study which shows that a family-based therapy strategy was impactful in helping the individuals recover quickly from treatment.

By treating the family as a whole, it can help the individual understand how the family's dynamic correlates to their binging. Be enthusiastic and involved as much as possible. You may need a lot of energy to be a constant support to these individuals so, make sure that you take care of your emotional health too. Also, be prepared for any kind of uncomfortable revelations about their weight, traumatic experiences, depression and childhood experiences.

The role of society and binge eating

Some of the current studies about eating disorders, in general, imply that these disorders are a combination of environmental and genetic factors. While environmental factors alone can't be held responsible for developing an eating disorder, the role of social pressure cannot be undermined when it comes to binge eating.

It can have a lasting impact on individuals who are genetically predisposed to developing eating disorders. For instance, in North America, both genders are told that in order to be successful and happy one need to be thin and fit.

So, each time they walk into a store, they look at skinny or beefy mannequins and aspire to be of the same shape. If that isn't enough, fashion magazines are full of images of muscular men and emaciated women on the front cover.

It may be surprising to know that thousands of women today are starving themselves to attain the ideal figure. This results in triggering their food cravings and their eating habits slowly start going downhill.

The Media

Clearly, the media has been a major influence in people's eating disorders. Most television shows feature super fit looking actors who have endured hours of intense workouts and starved themselves of proper nutrition in order to get into the skin of the character. Some have even resorted to breast implants, liposuction and other forms of plastic surgery.

It's as if society is brainwashing the youth into believing that being thin is a must if you want to be accepted. Teenagers and even adults spend a lot of time on social media platforms that promote self-comparison against an ideal body shape. As per a particular study[5], it has shown that spending excessive time on Facebook and binge eating are interlinked.

If we are constantly comparing ourselves to others we see on TV or social media, it can lead to feelings of low self-esteem and depression. As a way to cope with these emotions, we may engage in binge eating behavior. Often times it may feel as if we do not have control over the way we look, but we can control what we eat, when we eat and how much we eat. Having this level of control may be more rewarding and may distract our minds from the emotional pain caused by low self-esteem.

Diet Commercials

The diet ads that pop up on your computer screen or television send out a message that one can only be happy once they lose weight. While you are standing in the queue at the grocery store, you happen to glance the magazines, which claim to offer the best diet advice and instantly feel motivated to alter your dietary habits.

What you don't realize is that extreme diets can only make you fall into unhealthy patterns of food. We, as a society, spend billions of dollars every to get that perfect look, but fail to pay attention to what matters the most; food! The fashion and diet industries aren't completely to blame for society's obsession with an ideal figure.

We as humans need to start accepting each other for who we are and not how we appear to be.

Eight Habits That Make Binge Eating Worse

Here is a brief look at the eight habits you should stay away from in your fight against the binge eating disorder.

Not planning meals ahead of time

You can't wing it every time when it comes to your meals. There is a reason why your binge eating symptoms are getting worse, and the reason could be your lack of meal planning. If you are going about your meals in a haphazard manner, it's going to be difficult to control your cravings when they emerge.

When you don't carry home-packed meals, you are compelled to impulsively hog on any unhealthy item that is served in your office. If you don't find enough time to prepare your own meals, you can always order them from a restaurant that serves healthy food, but you will have to be extremely careful of your portions. And even ordering a meal from a restaurant almost every single day would need some planning.

Whatever you chose to do, just ensure that all your meals are predefined and that you aren't consumed by strong impulses to binge eat. If you have a busy week ahead, take out sometime on the weekends to figure out what and how much you will be eating throughout the next 5 days.

Don't miss a chance to pack any leftovers from your fridge. They will always come in handy when you skip your breakfast or miss your lunchtime.

Always suppressing your cravings

I mean seriously, don't give a cold shoulder to your cravings. Eating a tiny portion of the chocolate cake isn't going to make you binge eat. On the other hand, if you suppress a strong desire to indulge in some cheat meals, that's exactly what will make you binge on food later.

A lot of doctors suggest that you are better off attending to your cravings as soon as they arise. However, instead of emptying a tub full of ice cream, you should be consuming only a small portion of it. Another trick is to share that piece of chocolate cake or pizza slice with a friend. That way you wouldn't end up eating more than the share you planned to consume.

When you make a planned event out of your cravings, they won't come back to haunt you later. Instead of forcing yourself to resort to withdrawal or willpower when the craving comes at you with full force, a more sustainable response would be to allow yourself to make some indulgence. When you do this, you won't find yourself grumpy or frustrated anymore and that will help you be more relaxed, thereby giving you the ability to stop yourself from overeating.

Why Therapy Is So Important

Acceptance and commitment therapy (ACT) is an approach that has been empirically shown to support recovery in people with disordered eating. Just like the acronym suggests, this method involves taking action in order to change or recover. By taking action, as opposed to solely talking through your fears, you are able to more effectively challenge the fears and anxiety that have been holding you back. Most likely, these deeply rooted fears and anxiety began during childhood. As children, we have very few options to address our emotional pain. In order to get through discomfort when we were younger, we avoided it, acted out, or blamed ourselves and tried to fix it in some way.

To heal these damaging thoughts and behaviors, you must be willing to name the feelings you've avoided and experience them. This could mean reflecting and writing about them in a journal or using a voice or video recording or talking to someone supportive, such as a close friend or therapist. The second step is to allow the feelings to just be rather than judging, dismissing, or jumping to fix them. As you do so, trust that they will not last forever and accept them as they are. Unlike many external things in your life, these feelings cannot be controlled. When you stop trying to control or avoid feelings, the internal conflict that keeps you from moving through an emotion will subside.

The Benefits of a Support Group for Overeaters

Struggling with overeating can be a real challenge, and sometimes you might feel as if you are completely alone in your journey of trying to conquer your eating disorder. Although there are a lot of things that you can do on your own and with the help of a physician and nutritionist in order to become healthy again, you are missing out on the great opportunity to help yourself if you haven't attended a support group for overeaters. You can also join forums like BEAT for the UK and NEDA in the USA, where you can share with other people. Although there are some critics who don't like the idea of these programs, you will probably find that the benefits greatly outweigh the disadvantages and that a support group for overeaters might be just what you need to overcome your addiction.

Realize That You Aren't Alone

When you're hiding in your room and consuming as much food as you can possibly cram in your mouth and then deal with the aftereffects and guilt of doing so, you might feel as if you are the only one in the world who is going through these types of feelings. However, attending a support group for overeaters will allow you to see that there are other people from all walks of life who are dealing with the same types of problems that you are dealing with. This can help ease the feeling of being alone and can help you feel motivated to work on your issues.

Find Out the Causes of Your Eating Disorder

In order for you to start effectively working on repairing your disordered way of eating, you will have to understand what is causing you to do it in the first place. There are a lot of different factors that can contribute to causing someone to overeat, and sorting through these problems with others who have been where you are now can help you get the boost that you need.

Work on Your Emotional and Spiritual Self

Although overeating might seem like something that is purely physical, it usually stems from some sort of emotional or psychological issue. In an overeaters' support group, however, you can talk about and work on your emotional and spiritual self instead of just focusing on the physical things. This will give you the opportunity to feel better and tackle your eating disorder from the inside out instead of the other way around.

Make New Friends

It can be very difficult to form friendships and relationships with others when you are going through an eating disorder, especially if you feel as if no one whom you come into contact with actually understands you and the eating disorder that you are going through. Fortunately, however, you can make lots of great friendships in an overeaters' support group, and you won't have to worry about the people whom you come into contact not understanding you and what you are dealing with.

Get Support

Getting support from people who actually care about your disorder and who want to help you can work wonders for you and your recovery when you are finally ready to do something about your overeating, and you can get all the support that you need in an overeaters' support group. Not only will you be able to sit down and talk to understanding individuals about what you are going through, but you can also even get a sponsor whom you can contact any time that you need to talk to him or her about your problems. Having this support might be just what you need in order to tackle your overeating problem, and you will probably feel good in knowing that there are people out there who want to support you.

Figure Out a Plan

Overeaters' support groups do not usually advocate one specific diet or another; instead, they will encourage you to speak to your physician or with a nutritionist to come up with a plan that is right for you. However, the group will help you understand how important it is to quit overeating. They will help you determine how you have gotten to this point in the first place and what causes you to overeat. They can help you work on your inner self so that you and your doctor or nutritionist can come up with a plan for working on your outer self—your overeating.

Prevent Relapses

If you are someone who overeats, you have probably tried to quit doing so more times than you can count. However, you might have found it very hard to actually quit overeating and stay that way for good, especially without a good, strong support system. Luckily, however, a support group for overeaters can provide you with the encouragement and accountability that you need in order to tackle this disorder, which can help prevent you from relapsing and which can also help you get back on track in the event that you do make a few slipups during recovery.

Save Money

Although your health and well-being is certainly more important than any sum of money in the world, you might be concerned about the effect that the eating-disorder treatment will have on your wallet. Luckily, there are plenty of overeaters' support groups out there that are free to participate in, allowing you to get the help that you need without worrying about spending more than you can afford.

The Science Behind Emotional Eating

When overcoming binge eating disorders, it is important to look at the neurological reasons behind why people have them in the first place. When we are able to identify the causes, it is easier to see the effects. Then, we can look at that cause and try to minimize it, so it won't end up having as much of an effect as it might have before. I thought I was simply weaker than those who were able to stick to a strict diet and exercise routine. I figured I just hadn't found the right weightless supplement, or there was another diet like Atkins I just hadn't discovered yet. I never realized that I had an eating disorder and that I needed to discover the underlying neurological reasons behind the way I was feeling.

It is a very uncomfortable thing to deal with. The first reason it is so challenging for many is because of the need to confront your past trauma. It's never easy to go back and look at the things that caused you so much pain. Most of us would much rather pretend everything is okay and that we are fine with what we've been through. Admitting that something that happened to me as a child was still hurting me now made me feel weak. I felt like if I couldn't handle the experiences I'd gone through as a kid, I wouldn't be able to handle experiences as an adult. So, I just pretended everything was fine. Instead of dealing with it, we push it out of our mind, beginning a toxic cycle.

Body image becomes identity very quickly, especially for women. Eating disorders are more dangerous for men, since they will be much less likely to report that they have any issues with what they eat or their body image. However, women are still more likely to develop eating disorders as a result of trauma or mental illness, while men are have a higher chance of becoming addicted to drugs and alcohol.

For many women, especially young women, the type of body you have can be the type of person that you are, if you put an emphasis on body image. A woman that is very tall, slim, and sleek might look like a model, so more people will treat her like one and she'll feel that way herself. A woman full of curves, with a large butt and breasts might have a higher level of sex appeal for some people, making her seem more desirable. A woman who is overweight might be shamed because people think that she's lazy or gluttonous, so she will be treated that way and do the same for herself. Though body image is something that men have to deal with as well, the level this can impact young girls makes it especially challenging.

The Need for Control

One reason people will experience eating disorders is because they feel like they need to gain control in some form or another. I felt like I had no control over my life. Everything was stressful and overwhelming, and I thought I had to deal with it all on my own. I ended up turning to food to fulfill a need inside of me, but what I got instead was a dangerous eating disorder. Food was one thing I could control. I had the power to drive to McDonald's and get three cheeseburgers, and no one was around to stop me. I picked up the food and put it in my mouth. I had my car stocked with snacks. It made me feel powerful during a time when I felt truly helpless.

Those who look for control enjoy the power they get with emotional eating and other eating disorders. Especially for those that have body image issues, they feel as though their body is out of their control. Though you can dress a certain way or exercise and undergo surgery to alter your body, you still can't control how others perceive you. Some women with larger breasts talk about the struggle of being hypersexualized. Even in sweatshirts and baggy clothes, these women still feel uncomfortable with their shape, with many people perceiving them as sexy even though they are simply existing. When we live in a world where we feel like we have no control over our body, we will look for that power in other ways.

The reason we need control is simple: for survival. Everyone has control issues, it's just a matter of understanding the level of control you need. You need to feel like you are in charge of something in order to make you feel secure about your survival. You can't control if it rains, but you can control if you bring an umbrella. That's what we want. Just the assurance that we can take care of ourselves, and that we have enough control on our own.

It is important to not confuse control with power, either. Many people want control, but they don't necessarily want to be the president, or a police officer, or any other sort of influencer who holds power. We simply want the feeling, or illusion, that we have power. We want that desire to be fulfilled and will look to do it in many different ways.

Sometimes, we become insecure while struggling with perfectionism. Perfectionism doesn't mean that you want to be perfect, it just means that you have a hard time doing anything without consistently thinking about your flaws. Perfectionists won't always appear to have it all together. They will just struggle with simple tasks, like folding laundry or doing their hair, without getting caught up on all their perceived mistakes. Insecurity can stem from perfectionism, or vice versa. Either way, a low self-esteem is challenging, because you only look at your negative qualities and ignore all the things that are good.

Eating disorders are unhealthy, but sometimes, people think that what they're doing is good for them. Some feel as though they don't have a problem if they binge eat and then either purge themselves or go through starvation periods. It makes you feel strong. It is something that you are in charge of.

It is your identity, your thing that was special to you — a secret. Many people with eating disorders will also state that they don't necessarily enjoy the secret, but they find comfort in knowing that it is their own. It is knowledge only they have, and it comes from an intimate time when they are able to be alone.

You think that you are in control, but you are not. It becomes who you are. Though I was controlling what food I put in my mouth and how much, there was something inside of me that I couldn't control, which was telling me I needed to have it in the first place. I was in charge of getting the food, but my brain was enforcing my desire to get it in the first place. I had the illusion of power, which is what we crave the most.

Why We Choose Food

Inside our brains, we have opioid peptides. These neurotransmitters, which are also known as endorphins, are what helps give us good feelings. When you hear opioid, you might think of a drug like heroin. The reason why these types of drugs are so powerful is because they elicit those high endorphin feelings. Many things will get those opioid peptides active, and one of those things is sugar.

When you binge eat, you are overloading your brain with endorphins, especially because you are likely binging food that's high in sugar. Eventually, you build up an endorphin resistance, and your body will start to desperately crave those endorphins when they're not around. When your body experiences a chemical imbalance, it does whatever it thinks it should to balance that out. This is how addictions start.

Picture someone who was physically abused throughout their life, leading to complex PTSD, anxiety, and depression. Now, they drink every night in order to release the pain that comes along with dealing with that past trauma. Their brain balances out while they're drunk. The chemical imbalance isn't as intense as it was when they were sober during the day. However, when the alcohol fades, the imbalance comes back. So, the next day, they have to drink again. Our brains know they need to regulate our endorphin, cortisol, and other important hormone levels. Our brains also know how to find those balances- — but what they don't know, however, is how to achieve them in a healthy way. We will become addicted to things that give us that chemical balance, and food does that, especially when consumed in excess amounts.

When you are stressed out, your body releases cortisol. This is known as the stress hormone, because it is released by the liver during times when you are under a lot of pressure or holding onto great anxiety. Cortisol can be responsible for increasing your appetite — so, when you are stressed out, you are going to eat more simply because your appetite is much more intense.

We also choose food because it tastes good. There's no denying that eating a bowl of ice cream tastes way better than eating a leaf of kale. Sure, you might have moments where you'd certainly rather eat something healthy. We would all feel pretty sick, physically and mentally, if we ate cake for breakfast, pizza for lunch, and ice cream for dinner every day. Sounds like a great diet plan for my taste buds, but the older I get, the harder it is for me to eat nothing but unhealthy food. Still, I'd rather eat a bowl of ice cream than a kale salad when I have snack cravings, at least. I don't think I need to explain that sugar tastes better than healthy food. We know it, our kids know it, and even some animals are aware of this difference. What many of us don't know, however, is why sugar tastes so much better.

I remember being a teenager, lying in bed after eating cookies and candy, and wondering why I'd done that to myself. I had carrots, green peppers, strawberries, and other healthy food in the fridge that I could have eaten, but instead, I went right for the candy. Why did the candy have to taste so much better? Why couldn't the healthy stuff be what really tasted the best? Well, after doing a bit of research, I found out that a big reason is because we evolved from primates, who mostly ate sweet food, such as fruit from trees.

Our taste buds allow us to try new foods, so we are able to find the ones that will best satisfy our needs. Though you aren't aware of which foods are better for you based on taste alone, our ancestors were on a more animalistic level, which is why we have expanded our menus much more than when we were primates. If we didn't have taste buds, we would just eat one food, all day. Sticking to one food isn't healthy, however, because we wouldn't get all the nutrients and vitamins we actually need.

It is important to know how present sugar is in our foods, and that it doesn't just exist within cakes, candies, and ice creams. When you think of sugar, that is likely your first thought. However, most junk food is going to be high in sugar, as well. If you go through any fast food drive-thru and were actually provided with nutritional information, you find there's a high level of sugar in your burgers, even though they don't taste sweet like a desert.

Starches are forms of glucose that do not taste as sweet. This is why stuff like bread, pizza, mashed potatoes, and other high-starch foods taste so good but aren't very good for you. The most binge-able foods I ate were candy, cookies, ice cream, and cake. When I binged something savory, however, I would binge burgers, rolls, macaroni and cheese, and any and all forms of potatoes. Both of these categories of food are things that are high in sugar and can easily become addictive.

What to do When You Feel Stressed and Want to Eat Unnecessarily

When you feel like binging and remind yourself you can't, you will likely have a big feeling of frustration. Not only will you probably already be stressed, which is what caused the desire to binge, but you will also feel more stressed that you can't binge. In order to make these moments easier, you're going to have to find alternative methods of coping.

Listening to your body will be an important step. Sometimes, we might not even realize how to do that. For so long, we didn't listen to our bodies — instead, we just listened to our heads. Our stomachs would stretch and cause us pain, but that didn't matter, and we'd keep eating. Learn to listen to your body. When you want to eat, ask yourself if you're actually hungry or if it's stress.

The Emotions You Will Feel

The biggest emotion you'll feel in this journey is frustration. You're going to be mad that you can't eat. You're going to be mad about all the times you binge ate before, because if you hadn't been so unhealthy in the past, you could binge eat now (at least, that's what I told myself). You're going to be frustrated that you feel the need to binge, and you're going to be frustrated that your anger and impatience aren't going away.

Remember, all these feelings are valid. You are not wrong for having any single one of them. What could be wrong is what you decide to do with them.

Journal

When you are feeling stressed, grab your journal. Write down everything you're feeling and just let yourself freely express your emotions. This is also helpful because you can take this journal to therapy and give examples of your thought patterns when you aren't actually feeling them.

Another exercise you can do in your journal is to write a letter. Write a letter to yourself, or someone who made you angry. Write whatever you want in this letter, no matter how mean or nasty it might sound. Once you're done, destroy the letter. Tear it up, burn it, flush it down the toilet. When you are able to do that, you'll start to feel a lot better about the built-up emotions that you've been holding onto.

Go for A Walk

I used to hate going for walks. Any form of exercise was triggering for me, so I stayed inside as much as possible. After some encouragement from online friends and people around me, I realized I needed to give walking a try — and not power-walking with weights in my hands. Walking helps me to be mindful. I can take in my surroundings slowly and accept where I am, no matter how I might be feeling. Whenever I feel like binging, if it's really intense, sometimes I'll just leave my apartment. I won't bring any money with me either, so I can't grab a snack or anything else. The point of the walk is to help you work through your emotions and bring you back to a place where you're centered and peaceful.

Drink Water

You might have rolled your eyes pretty intensely when you read that. At any given time, if you Google "how to feel better," "how to lose weight," or "how to stop binge eating," drinking water is on every single one of those lists. Having a glass of water isn't going to cure any issues you have. but it will, however, make you feel less hungry.

I've also found that a lot of issues I have stem from being dehydrated. Headaches, backaches, and stomach pains can sometimes come simply from not drinking enough water, and you'll realize if you drink more water regularly, your overall mood will immensely improve.

Action Step #8

Buy a reusable water bottle and make it a habit to take it everywhere you go. Make sure it's one that's safe to reuse, and one that you won't easily lose. Personalize it with stickers or other decals if you want, but whatever you do, make sure that you have it by you at all times.

Ending Well and Beginning Again   "Problems" Are Opportunities

When you face a setback, take a moment to nondefensively and nonjudgmentally learn from the setback. A scientific way to change behavior in this nonjudgmental spirit is through behavior analysis. In this systematic approach, you specify a behavior you wish to modify, determine the causes of the behavior, and identify the potential challenges in implementing change. Instead of approaching a problem by fast-forwarding through it or avoiding facing it, which obscure detail, think of this method as hitting pause. Slowing down, you carefully examine the intricacies of factors underlying your behavior—external events, emotions, thoughts, and sensations—to gather important information that will help you move forward (Linehan 1993a). You can do this examination right away after a setback or at a later time when you have some perspective.

As an example of using behavior analysis, let's say you are repeatedly late. You can either get caught in shame and worry about this or use that same mental energy to thoroughly uncover the factors in the behavior. (In this case it might be best to notice the nuances related to this behavior once you're settled at work rather than as you run through the door, panic-stricken.) When you slow down and deliberately examine the behavior, you might note the following events, actions, and circumstances:

- Felt anxious and went to bed late

- Hit the snooze button

- Had the thought "It's okay if I'm a little late"

- Checked e-mail

- Spent time making wardrobe choices

- Noticed feeling fat and thought, "Changing clothes won't take long"

- There was a line at the café where I buy coffee

- Saw my old friend at the café and stopped to talk

- Thought, "It's rude to rush away"

- Uncomfortable shoes slowed my pace

- Caught in traffic

In slowing down to notice the details, you generate more potential solutions than the overly simple "I shouldn't hit the snooze button." Upon reflection, you may notice such possible choices as:

- Reduce vulnerability by getting more sleep

- Cope ahead and choose outfit the night before

- Notice thoughts

- Surf urges to check e-mail

- Practice mindfulness around time

- Problem solve: explore alternate routes to work; build in more time; buy espresso machine

If you were to combine several of these solutions, you might really change your timing.

Catch Yourself Capitulating

One propensity you may notice is the urge to *capitulate*, or give in to a behavior, such as using food to cope, overeating, not accepting, or moving away from what you care about. Capitulating is not passive—it's actively deciding not to bother (Safer, Telch, and Chen 2009). For example, if you notice that you haven't lost weight and feel sad, you may think, "It's too late," or, "Screw this," and head over to your favorite bakery. Capitulating is really different from acceptance. It's willful and comes from emotion mind. What happens when you repeatedly capitulate? You may come to believe you "can't" or feel hopeless. In noticing that capitulating is a choice, you may bring awareness to urges, thoughts, feelings, and your values when you face a desire to capitulate. This moment is an opportunity to build a sense of resilience and mastery. You may keep track of the urge to capitulate in your behavior analyses.

Monitor What Matters to You

As this book comes to an end, what are your aspirations? If you were to set goals and practice coping ahead, how might you proceed? Purposefully pursuing your values requires commitment and a good plan. We've covered many concepts and explored many tools to employ. With so much new material, one of the most helpful methods to practice paying attention and building mastery is to keep track of what you did and how it went—mindfully, nonjudgmentally, and in a spirit of acceptance.

The goal here isn't to feel better or feel negative emotions less. In fact, you may feel negative emotions more as you practice awareness and acceptance. The goal is to live the valued life you chose. Achieving this will most likely mean you will be noticing—and keeping track of—both negative emotion and skillful action.

Many people find it difficult to remember events or emotions in detail. And in emotion mind it's also hard to consider all of the practices you've learned. Using a reminder list of tools learned and keeping track of using skills will help boost your practice.

There is also space for writing a brief general note on your day. As you self-monitor, notice and implement changes to practice moving toward your goals. For example, if you notice an instance of emotional eating, rather than beating yourself up, conduct a compassionate behavior analysis.

I warmly encourage you to try your best in experimenting with keeping track of what you choose. Do it for a while to see whether practicing these steps enriches your experience.

If the number of skills feels overwhelming, break it down: highlight five skills of your choice. You may also start at the beginning of the book, focusing on one or two skills to practice regularly and continuing to add a skill each week.

Monitoring will allow you to notice in detail how much you used a skill and also keep track of the intensity of your experience.

Each moment—and each day, and each week—is a chance to start again by accepting yourself more. Valued living is a lifelong journey that requires understanding and diligence, but the road is always right before your feet. There's no prerequisite for beginning and no punishment for faltering; we only begin, and begin again.

Exercise: Keeping Track of Skills Used

For each day of the week, take note of what skills you used. In the chart below, the names of some skills are followed by a word or two of guidance that will help you usefully describe your use of the skill. It may also help you to use numbers when noting which skills you used and how useful they were, as follows:

0 = Didn't think about or use

1 = Thought about, didn't use

2 = Tried to use but couldn't

- 3 = Used skill; not helpful

- 4 = Used skill; found somewhat helpful

- 5 = Used skill; found very helpful

	Mon	Tues	Wed	Thurs	Fri	Sat	Sun
Notice and Label Emotions (specify emotions and intensity on a scale of 1–10)							
Accept Emotions							
Practice Willingness							
Notice Emotional Eating (specify when and where)							
Practice Mindfulness							
Formally:							
Informally:							
Mindful Eating							
Breakfast:							
Lunch:							
Dinner:							
Snacks:							

	Mon	Tues	Wed	Thurs	Fri	Sat	Sun
Eat at Moderate Hunger, Stop at Moderate Fullness							
Notice Mind States (emotion, reasonable, wise)							
Reduce Vulnerability							
Add Positives:							
Build Mastery:							
Cope Ahead:							
Notice and Surf Urges							
Observe Thoughts and Catch Interpretations							
Distress Tolerance: Review Costs and Benefits							

	Mon	Tues	Wed	Thurs	Fri	Sat	Sun
Soothe							
One Moment at a Time:							
With Other Senses:							
Find Meaning:							
Contribute:							
Self-Compassion							
Notice Critical Thoughts:							
Practice Loving-kindness:							
Ask Clearly:							
Focus on Higher Values							
Notice AIBs							
Catch Capitulating							

Notes

Mon	
Tues	
Wed	
Thurs	
Fri	
Sat	
Sun	

A Step-by-Step Guide to Eating Intelligently

If we want to live, then we have to eat. However, eating smart and healthy is something we need to train ourselves to do, especially in this day and age. Eating intelligently requires becoming conscious about what we eat.

We all know that what we eat and our health are in sync. The latter won't be possible without the former. Maintaining maximum health depends on what goes in through our mouths. Through what you eat, you take control of your life. Intelligent eating is a proactive measure with positive results. It's something that becomes a part of you, as you make the right choices one day at a time. Your body will thank you for it, and you'll be glad you decided to do this!

Eating intelligently is not about dieting in a particular way. It is modifying your normal eating habits for a better way of life. Intelligent eating, unlike some dietary plans, is a long-term project intended to maximize one's health and reduce the chances of illnesses. What I'm trying to say is I'm not offering you a weight loss program. I'm offering you the tools you need to improve the state of the mind and body. Intelligent eating is for people who are really interested in improving their health.

Quality Over Quantity

We must have heard constantly that food gives us energy and energy is required for us to be able to carry out our day to day activities. Eating intelligently requires a calculated approach at nourishment. You have to be able to eat well without eating too much or too less. You have to be able to eat at the right time without having to fast or skip meals.

Because, it takes a lot to be able to balance the right amount of fats, carbs, proteins and vitamins in a meal, after all, you can't go around carrying a scale. Everyone would doubt your sanity, you weirdo! Just kidding.

Your Brain and Glucose

Where food is concerned, the brain can be very selective. Like a petulant five year old with a sweet tooth, it loves simple sugar molecules. It loves glucose to be exact. And when the brain isn't provided with the glucose it needs, it gets really cranky and annoyed.

Since our bodies can easily produce glucose by breaking down carbohydrates, it would be right to conclude limiting carbs could reduce or impair cognitive function, right? Wrong. Your brain can actually function perfectly well on *ketones,* which are a byproduct of broken down fat. Some would argue it's even cleaner fuel for your brain, but this book isn't about that. The point is carbs are important, even if everyone wants to give them a bad rep. Just be sure to get the good sort in your belly! That means rather than have a burger or a bagel, you can opt for some whole wheat bread, or choose to have some wholegrain cereal other than the one that orange tiger Tony keeps pushing.

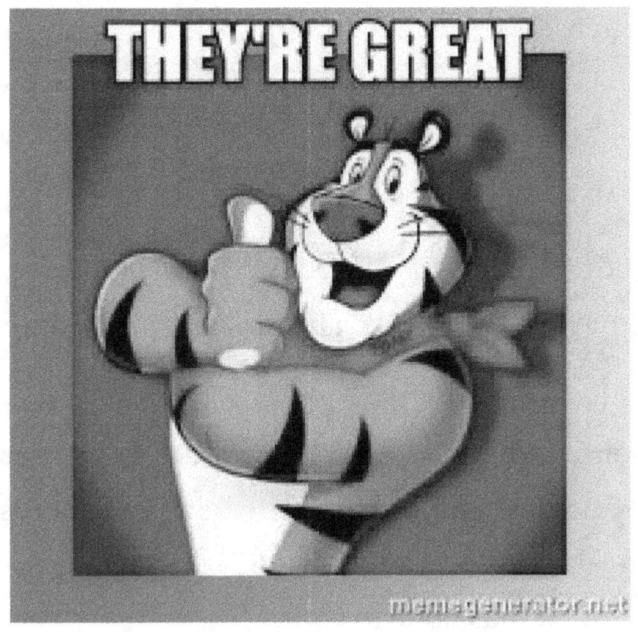

They're NOT!

Give your body the right stuff to work with, and you gradually stop craving all the bad stuff. Did you know the less sugar you take in, the less you crave? In fact, after long enough, it starts to taste just wrong!

So we're talking about eating intelligently, right? What would be the intelligent thing to do when you get a craving for cocaine's cousin Sugar? *Opt for foods with natural sugar in them.* Natural sugar is very good for our brains. Try as much as possible to include them as part of a balanced diet, with your meals, daily.

The Benefits of Intelligent Eating

There is so much to gain from fueling your body intelligently.
You feel better, for starters. Your body's like a finely tuned
engine. What do you think is going to happen if you fuel a
Ferrari with Monster, instead of actually gas? Yeah, you can say
goodbye to that 'rari now. It's gone.

The same thing applies to your body! If you wouldn't put the
wrong fuel in your car, why treat your body any different or less!

When you give your body the right foods, when you choose to
eat intelligently, what happens? You start to feel better. You
start to *look better*. Your body is better able to fight disease, and
to repair the damage all that junk food feasting powered by
emotional hunger has done to you.

You get maximum energy. You're less bloated, and you have way
less flatulence than you used to. If you suffer from Irritable
Bowel Syndrome, the symptoms are lessened significantly.

Listen to Your Body Talk

No, I'm not talking about body language in conventional terms. I
mean **pay attention to what your body is telling you.**
Have you noticed that every time you drink something that has
dairy in it, you tend to break out and you have horrible stomach
cramps? *Then quit taking dairy for a bit.* Maybe a couple of
weeks. Try it after the break, and if you notice you get the exact

same reaction, guess what? You're lactose intolerant! So let go of the milk, and find other delicious alternatives.

Do you find you feel absolutely terrible every time you overeat? Aren't you sick of that? Listen, the only reason you feel that way is *because your body does not like that!* So what's the intelligent thing to do in this scenario? You could

- Chew slower
- Chew deliberately
- Put your fork down in between chews
- Sip some water every couple of minutes

Basically do anything to slow you down! This way, your brain is able to realize when you're full *before* you've eaten so much you look like Santa Claus.

Before you decide what to eat, ask your body! Does this sound weird? Well, you'd better try this. If you pay close attention, you'll realize you have certain cravings. Personally, when I get hungry, when I stop to ask myself that question, I might find I want a chicken salad. Then that's what I for. Your body is always speaking, if you'll listen.

Other times, I might randomly decide to have some snack, but then when I ask myself, "Yo Aron, buddy, are you actually hungry?" I realize there's a huge chance I'm just bored. Then I remember all the stuff I have to do, or stuff I do for leisure, and I go do that instead.

So don't be in a hurry to grab a bite to eat. Listen! And even if you think you really, really want a pizza, slow down and ask yourself, "What else would taste just as good and be twice as healthy?" If you can't figure it out, Google it! Whatever you do, slow down and take your time when it comes to food.

Change The Channel

Eating intelligently means not falling for every stupid advert you see on TV. Companies shell out millions and millions of dollars, year after year, just to get you to buy something. They have experts who are dedicated to figuring out the best way to manipulate your psychology. They want to manipulate you into reaching for your phone and making a call to your favorite burger or pizza joint, and they know ads are effective. Why?

When you're watching TV, your brainwaves are in alpha mode. In this state, you are highly suggestible. So after they've got you in that state of mind with whatever mindless drivel is on, guess what happens next! Ads!

If you have to watch your favorite show, make sure to skip these ads. Change the channel!

These industries do not give a flying fig about you, they just want to make their money, so, they will tell you anything to sell you their product. I think it's very telling their CEOs and executives won't even eat their own products all that often, if at all. What does that tell you? Think!

Trick Yourself

Here's something I did when I was a tad overweight from all that emotional eating, and badly needed to change my life and lose the pounds.

First, I wrote down every single food I knew was my weakness. The pizzas, the burgers, the chocolates, **everything.** A perfect little list of all my little temptations.

Next, beside each item, I wrote out some other healthy food that had the same mouth feel as the unhealthy stuff. Ice cream? No. Yogurt. Chips? No. Homemade, natural popcorn made in a pot, not in the microwave. That sort of thing. Soda? No. Sparkling water.

What did I do after that? I made a commitment to myself I would never use those words - the unhealthy foods - ever again. Not when speaking, and not when thinking. So when I'd start craving a soda, I'd say, "Man, I'm really craving sparkling water." You get it?

After a while, guess what happened? **I actually started to believe myself!** I believed I really did want water. I really did want carrots. I really did want fruit.

Another trick I played on myself was saying, "I don't eat THIS." So when I'd see something I liked that was pure junk, I'd remind myself gently, "I DON'T eat this." Not "can't," but DON'T. The distinction is important. It tells my subconscious mind, hey, this is good looking and all but it really isn't my thing. Guess what happens when you program your subconscious with the right messages? It begins to act accordingly!

Things You Can do to Improve Your Health and Cut Down on Emotional Eating

- ***Water! And more water!***

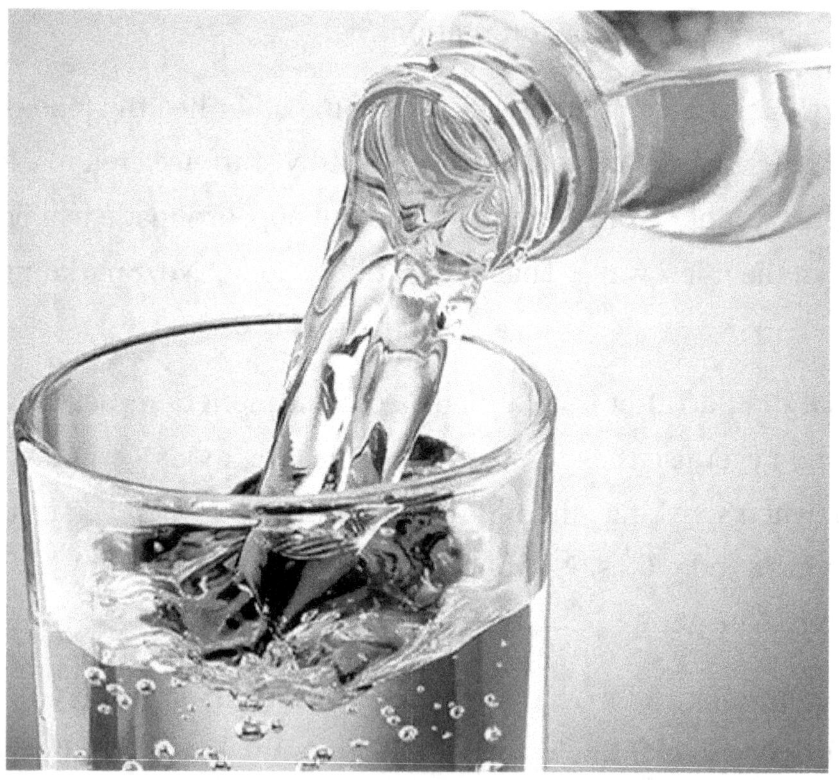

Feel hungry? First have a glass of water. Still feel hungry? Have another glass. If you're still hungry, then fine, go eat something! Even if you choose junk, you won't have enough room for it.

Staying hydrated is very important for your body's daily function. But many people do not drink enough. About 60 percent of our body is made up of water and that water is used up in transpiration (sweating), transportation of substances etc. And as regularly as it is used up, it also needs to be replaced. For all of you looking for flawless skin without having to buy expensive cosmetic products, water will really help you. It hydrates the skin and helps in the removal of dead skin cells.

Keeping hydrated also helps regulate the body's temperature. So, whenever you feel flushed, just drink a glass of water! It also helps control our blood pressure, and you will be less likely to suffer from a stroke or high blood pressure.

Water aids in the digestion of food and in so doing, helps burn a lot of calories, which research has shown helps a person lose belly fat.

There are a lot of suggestions in the media these days, on how much water a person should consume in a day. But doctors' advice is to stay very hydrated as the health benefits are many and as such have suggested that a person consume at least half a gallon of water in a day.

Don't fret, you don't have to finish it all in one go.

We know how our stomachs seem to slosh from one side to another when we drink too much water. It's not a particularly pleasant feeling. It's actually a real concern for a person not to drink **too much** water. Drinking too much water, too fast, within a short period of time causes our sodium levels to drop too low, which causes water intoxication or hyponatremia.

So you could be "drunk" on water.

- Fruits! And more Fruits!

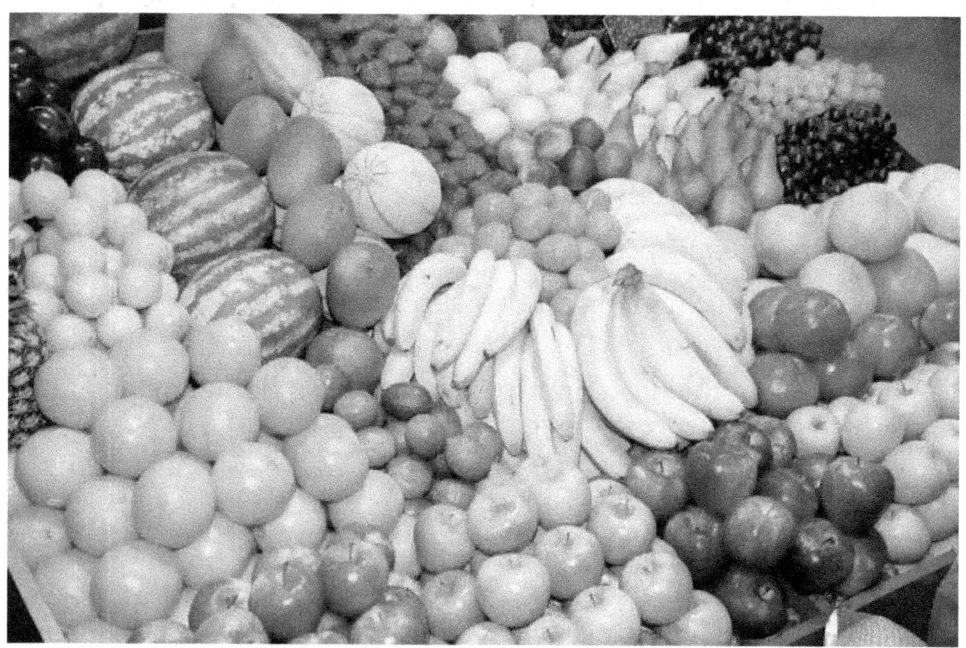

I am sure we have all heard the old saying, an apple a day keeps the doctor away. It's very true, in the literal sense.

Fruits are naturally low in fat content, carbs and calories but are rich in vitamins. Many fruits are the origin of important nutrients and are not eaten enough. Nutrients such as folic acid, potassium, citric acid and dietary fibre.

Fruits help boost our immune system and gives us a fighting chance against some consuming enough fruits can help reduce our chances of getting heart diseases, elevated blood pressure, even some cancers. *Amazing, right?*

Fruits are vitamin rich foods that help keep our energy levels up. Eating a good amount of fruits is healthy as long as it is part of a healthy diet plan. A fruit-only diet can be dangerous to the health because fruits are rich in natural sugar. If they are over consumed, your blood sugar levels might be elevated to an insanely dangerous height.

If you can squeeze in a small plate of fruit salad after dinner instead of your usual cream filled pastry for dessert, trust me, you will be better for it.

- *Exercise!* Move it, move it!

How many times have you watched people engaging in rigorous exercises and you know in your heart of hearts that no matter how much you tried or wanted to, you could never do what they are doing? *I mean, they make it look so simple!*

Their bodies seeming sculpted or honed from pure steel. Beautiful bodies with defined abs. But you are just watching them with your *generous* body. Not fat, *generous*.

You can always remedy that. It doesn't take much. You do not need all those fancy instruments of torture they have at the gym or go under the surgical knife. All you need is your will and a little bit of time.

Try running. It is a cardiovascular exercise. Popularly called "cardio." Why? Because it elevates your heart rate. *Running causes your heart to race!* It is a very healthy exercise that helps build and define muscles. It also helps strengthen our bones, because, during the course of the exercise our bones are made to bear the weight of our body, so they grow stronger so as to be able to withstand the constant pressure they get from being jolted.

Running also helps us stay in the healthy weight range, and helps shed some weight.

It also helps our respiration. When we run we burn energy and use up a lot of oxygen. That is why we breathe faster while running. Breathing fast causes us to unconsciously inhale faster, which causes our body to increase the production of oxygen and removal of carbon dioxide.

Many people have also said running helps them think better. And it helps them deal with emotions such as anger, hurt or annoyance. It can even help you feel less lethargic! Fancy that!

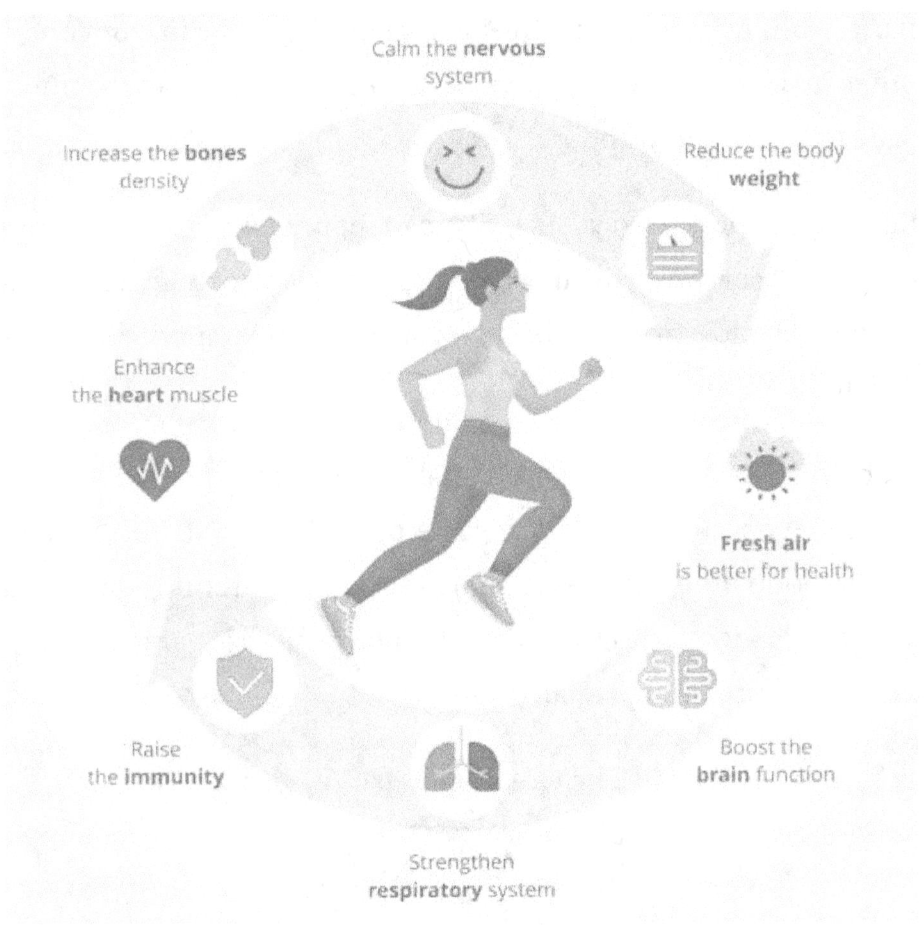

When I say running, I don't mean for you to take part in the Olympics, or run 20 miles every day. You could easily run from one end of your street to the other. You don't have to be as fast as Usain Bolt. Go at your own pace. It may be very difficult if you push yourself too hard, especially if it's something you are not particularly used to doing.

Try walking. We all walk, from the car to the house, the local store and back. We may even take a leisurely walk through the park. Walking is just the movement of our legs, one in front of the other in a pattern. You can do that, can't you? Just a 30-minute walk a day can do wonders!

Such a simple physical activity can help burn an impressive amount of calories. If you can dedicate at least forty five minutes of your time to a brisk walk daily, you will begin to noticeably lose weight in no time.

Like running, walking also helps our cardiovascular and pulmonary system. Walking also helps us develop stronger bones and to hone lithe muscles for a better body figure. It reduces our chances of developing a stroke or heart disease, and helps us maintain our blood pressure.

- Eat All The Green Things! Veggies for the Win!

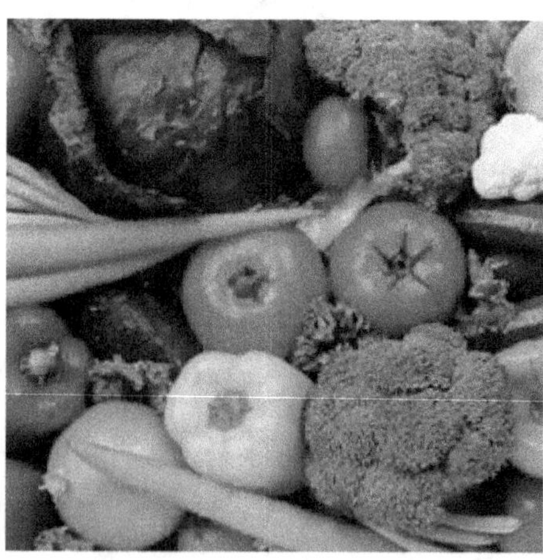

And the other stuff.

Vegetables are plants edible to humans. The word is used to classify all parts of an edible plant, including the stem, the root, the flower, the fruit, the seeds and the leaves. There are many different types of vegetables, but the point is to incorporate as many as possible in your meal without being wasteful.

It has been discovered that people who eat enough vegetables and fruits as part of their diet have a reduced risk of having chronic diseases. Vegetables are rich in various nutrients like; vitamins A, E and C, dietary fibre, potassium, and folic acid.

Vegetable diets Help reduce the risk of type-2 diabetes, coronary diseases (heart), stroke, high blood pressure, etc.

- Go to Sleep!

We are all well aware of what sleep is. It is something our body needs to be able to function properly. *Sleep* is a state of oneness between the body and the mind which takes place several hours every night, daily. It's a state in which the nervous system is at rest, the eyes are shut and all the muscles in the body are relaxed and our consciousness is temporarily suspended, until our waking moment, where consciousness is regained.

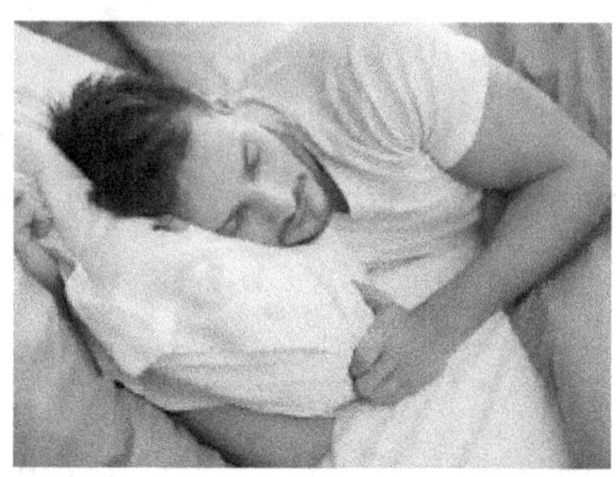

Sleep helps you relieve stress. Maybe after a long day job, after a bout of vigorous exercising, or when you are just bummed out. It also helps reduce depression. Maybe you are feeling depressed over having lost your job, losing a very much needed deal, being broke or watching your favorite team lost the match, a good night's sleep will go a long way. A lot of people have said they tend to feel more alert on waking up. Some even say they tend to remember things they might have forgotten during the day after a good night's rest.

Sleep is a very important part of our lives, there is no way around it. Did you know the less sleep you get, the more likely you are to binge eat when you wake up? So get some good, quality sleep. Don't stare at any screen for an hour before bed. Keep your room nice, dark, and at a cool, comfortable temperature. Invest in good pillows and a solid mattress. It will make all the difference to the quality of your sleep. I promise

If you follow all these tips, what you'll find is that you're going to have more of a handle on your emotional hunger. You'll find your dedication to following these steps will actually spill over, and give you the willpower you need to tell yourself you're not going to have another Twinkie.

Lapse Prevention

With the mind ruminating on automatic obsessive thoughts, we are vulnerable to a lapse, or a re-lapse. *A lapse is a one-time misstep, after which you correct your actions and remain committed to your recovery goals. A re-lapse is when you consciously refuse to try anymore, and stop "starting over."* Research shows that there are three high-risk situations that are associated with about 75% of all lapses. Those three situations are: (1) Situations where the person is experiencing a negative or painful emotional state, such as anxiety, depression, boredom, loneliness, or emptiness (2) Situations involving conflict with someone (3) Social pressure from others to drink/use, either direct or subtle.

Pre-determining your risky situations and developing a plan of action ahead of time to manage them greatly reduces the probability of a lapse. Triggers don't have to be really big things; in fact, the every-day variety can be just as difficult to manage. 75% of all lapses occur within the first 90 days of abstinence. 93% occur within the first 6 months following abstinence. Slips lead to future slips, and regular slips lead to relapse. The early stages of recovery are a time of high vulnerability.

A key factor in overcoming addictive behavior is becoming very proficient at self-soothing and calming techniques. To avoid relapse, carefully identify your triggers and "high risk" situations. When the craving begins, try to interrupt the destructive thought-cycle by applying the following self-soothing techniques:

Self-Intervention Exercise:

Cognitive Diffusion

Rather than suppressing, denying or ignoring the cravings, sit for a minute and write out what your mind is telling you. This technique is called, "Cognitive Diffusion," and means that you observe thoughts without judging them or having to obey them. The key is to remember that our thoughts aren't always true, which means you can dispute them. If you can't dispute them, at least inspect them! You simply want to tune in and listen to them, which can sometimes defuse the need to act on the thought. Observe them with a curious but detached awareness.

Example: "My thoughts are telling me to go have a cigarette again. They are telling me I can't manage how I will feel if I don't. They are telling me I need one, instead of want one."

Write out an example of what your mind might say to you when it begins to crave:

Self-Intervention Exercise:

Urge-Surfing

This is a meditation-based method of re-directing your "triggered self," and is mainly utilized in Dialectical Behavioral Therapy (DBT). Having the ability to psychologically "shift gears" is a core coping and self-soothing skill. Breathing through the craving (called Urge Surfing) is a method to respond vs. react, and can, with practice, interrupt the addictive cycle. By focusing your full attention on the craving sensations rather than suppressing them, denying what is happening or ignoring it, your ability to tolerate strong anxiety and to self-sooth will grow.

Procedure: The next time you're triggered, find a comfortable spot to sit or recline. Feel how tense and uptight your craving body feels. Don't resist experiencing the "awfulness of the moment." Remember, whatever you resist persists. You're going to get re-focused now on relaxing the body so your thoughts will relax in turn. Close your eyes if it helps you concentrate on your body, and breathe deeply. As you breathe in, your abdomen should rise. This is called "tummy-breathing." On the out-breath your abdomen should fall. If your tummy isn't going in and out, you are "shoulder breathing," which is a shallow type of breathing, what we normally do when we are tense. To aid in getting relaxed, think the word: "in," on the in-breath, and "out" on the out-breath. After your breathing has steadied, and you're beginning to feel in touch with your breath, repeat the word: "Relax. Relax. Re-laaaax," to yourself.

As you breathe through the sensation of craving (called Urge-Surfing), the cravings should diminish in intensity because you are redirecting your focus from your thoughts to your breath and body. It's a lot like breathing through birth contractions, called Lamaze Breathing. This mindfulness-based intervention can enable you to develop the ability to tolerate strong emotion. Using this craving-tolerance technique regularly (on a daily basis) can break the chain of addictive thinking, because it interrupts and re-directs the automatic compulsive thought from an uptight mind to a relaxed body.

Exercise Summary

1. When triggered remind yourself, "It's time for "Urge Surfing."

2. Acknowledge how tense your muscles and mind are by tuning into your body. Your body may feel: tense, tight, wiry, stiff, sweaty or cold, and you may have muscle agitation. Your mind may feel panicked, desperate, afraid, anxious, confused, etc.

3. Repeat the word, "Relax. Relax. Re-laaaax." Continue to repeat the word while Urge-Surfing.

4. After repeating the word, "Relax," get focused ONLY on your breathing.

5. As you breathe in your abdomen should rise, and on the out-breath it should fall. Think the word: "in," on the in-breath, and "out" on the out-breath. Some people like to put their hands on

their abdomens so they can "feel" their breathing, and check to see if they are doing it correctly.

6. Urge Surfing is difficult, especially at first. It's normal to feel disappointed because you may think you're not able to resists the craving for very long. However, the more you practice your "surfing skills," the better surfer you'll become. The goal is to RIDE THAT WAVE until you feel significant relief from the craving. Imagine you are in labor, breathing through contractions.

7. Example: If you Urge Surfed for 2 minutes the first time you tried it, you should be proud! You can keep a log of Urge Surfing times, so when you do it again, you can shoot for surpassing your own record. Tracking Urge Surfing builds confidence in your ability to cope with and manage cravings.

Self-Intervention Exercise:

Awareness of Universal Connection

This is a spiritual exercise which can be practiced anytime, anyplace:

1. Focus your attention on where your body touches an object (chair, bed, floor, desk, your clothes, etc.)

2. Consider the function of that object; how it serves you, what the object does for you.

3. Experience the subtle feelings of touching that object (i.e., it feels secure, it feels strong, it feels comfortable, it feels reassuring, etc.)

4. Touch and explore the object, considering all of its physical properties (it is smooth or hard, round or square, cold or warm, etc.)

5. Consider how you as a human being you are continually supported and protected by your environment. Realize that you are connected to all things in your environment, and all things are here for your maintenance, support and nurturance. Realize that consciousness is in you, just as it is (in some form) in the object. Realize you are both nourished by the sun, the air, the rain and the earth.

Write a statement of gratitude which arises in your heart for being cared for and supported by your environment:

If you can, imagine what this object might say to you, and write it in your notebook:

Choose from these sure-fire solutions when you feel yourself "losing grip" on your recovery goals:

A. Emergency Coping List (ECL) - When regular coping methods aren't effective, call all of the people on your ECL, and talk to the first person who calls you back. Now is not the time to be choosey, be grateful for any support. Make sure you tell whoever is on your ECL that should they get a call from you, you're going to need their support. Add such people as: group therapy members, AA sponsors, as well as supportive friends and family.

B. Safety Zone - Get into your mental safety zone by creating a comforting environment for yourself. Change into your comfiest clothes, get a blanket, hold a treasured item, lock your doors, take a soothing bath, hide in your bed, turn the lights on or off, hold or talk to your pet, but change your environment in some way, i.e. letting cool air in or warming up the house. Next, imagine a favorite place in your mind. Allow yourself to go there, and stay there as long as you can. Take a "mini-mental vacation" and visualize being completely free of the worry in your special place.

C. Remove Triggers - If there is something in your environment which is tempting you to have a lapse, remove it from your environment. This may mean you'll have to get up and go somewhere else, or it may mean you'll have to remove the item, ask the people to leave, or hang up the phone. Remind yourself that if you fail to confront your triggers, you're on a slippery slope.

D. Coping List - Write out a Coping List from the suggestions below, and add your own ideas to the list. Healthy coping activities can distract you when you feel the familiar tug of old patterns. Keep the list in a common area where you'll see it regularly.

Healthy coping includes: Routines, healthy meals, plenty of sleep, exercising, sex, self-intervention exercises, group therapy, individual therapy, recreation and socialization, reading inspiring and motivational s, asking for support from people who care when stressed or tempted, self-forgiveness, and expressing your creativity.

Negative coping includes: Blaming others, blaming ourselves, justifying our behavior or making excuses, over-indulging, seeing only the bad in ourselves, risk-taking behaviors, reacting emotionally or impulsively, or acting-out.

1. Urge Surf-Relax, belly breath and meditate on your breath as you think: "in" and "out"

2. Call a family member or friend for support

3. Exercise-Go to the gym, exercise at home or take a walk for some air and to clear your head

4. Read Positive Affirmations

5. Do something creative-music, writing, art, dance

6. Think about a healing color: imagine yourself bathed in it, strengthened by it

7. Call on your Higher Power or Higher Self for guidance

8. Listen to music that you enjoy

9. Take a soothing bath

10. Allow yourself to cry

11. Cook

12. Read a book, magazine

12. Watch TV or a movie (especially a funny one)

13. Repeat words of an affirmation as you take a walk

14. Remind yourself it will pass, and repeat the word, "Relax. Relax. Re-laaaax."

15. Journal your feelings

16. Visualize yourself as a tree, roots firmly planted in the ground and immobile

17. Carry a stone in your pocket which you rub, that reminds you to surrender your worries when you touch it

18. Get a massage; get a manicure or pedicure, or a hair cut

19. Record your experiences and feelings in a small recorder

20. Treat yourself to a meal or dessert out

21. Repeat words to a song over and over

22. Color with crayons (my personal favorite)

23. Take a much-needed nap

24. Buy yourself flowers or some other token of self-love and appreciation

25. Light a candle in honor of your achievements, and in faith for the healing yet to come

26. Practicing awareness while washing the dishes-Wash dishes and contemplate each dish as an object of contemplation. Do not hurry: consider the dishes, each dish as sacred.

27. Practicing awareness while cleaning house-Slowly move and fully focus your attention on each task. If your mind wanders from "being in the moment" of the task, bring your awareness

back to your breath, and focus on your breath until you are able to re-focus back to your awareness of cleaning

28. Options List-In any situation, you have choices. Make a list of all the options you can think of

29. Get organized-You'll feel more "in control" through to-do lists and a clean environment

30. Structure your day-An active schedule keeps you productive and connected to others

31. Detach from emotional pain-Distract, walk away, and change the "channel"

32. Identify the belief-What unconscious negative belief have you been ruminating on?

E. Just for Today Agreement - When you are in a downward spiral, sometimes the only thing that can save us from a lapse is to "be our word" to ourselves. Although our own promises to ourselves and others may have been compromised many times in the past, in a moment of psychological crisis, write out a brand new agreement, one that is new and fresh, and then read it over many times until the feelings of crisis pass.

For example: "For today, I agree that I will: follow my smoking cessation plan, just for today.

I may not like it, I may even hate it, but I agree to do it just for today. I remember these feelings will pass, they will not last. I agree to this because: I want to feel proud of myself for conquering the urge."

Just for Today Agreement
(fill in the blanks)
"For today, I agree that I will: _______________________________,
just for today.

I may not like it, I may even hate it, but I agree to do it for today.

-and-

I remember these feelings will pass, they will not last.

I agree to this because: _______________________________."

What Do You Really Need?

Your primitive brain, as a result of survival drives resident in the amygdala, labors tirelessly to ensure that you meet your basic needs, one of which is the need for food.

We have seen how it endeavors to cause you to substitute food for any emotional lack or distress and even creates negative emotional affect and anxiety on its own to attempt to compel you to eat.

But in addition to your need for food, water, air to breathe — your basic needs — you also have higher needs which, if not met, will cause you emotional distress and can impair the quality of your life.

Your deeper needs include the need for love and compassion, social connection and feeling supported, peace and a connection with nature, creativity and a sense of control, and spiritual harmony.

You now have the ability to consciously control your prefrontal – amygdala interactions so that, rather than succumbing to the primitive brain's urgings and engaging in emotional eating, you can influence the primitive brain, soothing it and quieting its voice so that you can ignore it.

By mastering EEESY™ you are now master of your primitive brain.

Emotional eating is no longer something in which you will engage, but the urge arising from your primitive brain to eat when you are emotionally distressed will prove to be very useful.

We are now going to look at how you can discover the deepest needs which you lack in your life so that you can set about to meet them.

Not only will you, by doing this, stop your emotional eating at its source, but you will improve the quality of your life at a foundational level.

Before we proceed further, it is helpful to distinguish the difference between a need and desire.

There is no clear demarcation, once we have transcended our basic survival needs. However, we may define the difference between a need and desire in this way: a need is something which, if we fail to meet, we experience a fundamental impairment in our ability to function as humans.

In contrast, a desire is something which, although we may be able to survive perfectly well without it, we may not thrive, or at least not do as well as we could.

As an example, we have a need to live somewhere where we can have social interactions, be engaged productively, and have access to sufficient recreational opportunities to remain healthy and active.

But we may have a desire to live somewhere sunny.

Our needs may be met, but once we decide that we are solar powered and truly desire to live somewhere where we can enjoy sunshine year-round, we will have our best chance at thriving if we can move to a sunny locale.

The fact that your primitive brain is urging you to eat contrary to your eating plan, to engage in emotional eating, is indicative of something wrong in your life.

Something isn't right.

But what? How do you determine, with any degree of certainty, what is wrong?

To do this, you must first look at your emotional triggers.

To determine the need which you are failing to meet, you must first look at the nature of the emotional trigger.

When you experience the urge to eat contrary to your predetermined eating plan you'll use EEESY™ to avoid emotional eating.

But also note what emotional trigger caused your primitive brain's survival drives to engage.

Do this once you are sufficiently soothed from using your soothing food alternative of choice. Ask yourself, "What was I upset about?"

You may determine, for example, that your emotional trigger was a tough day at work caused by an unappreciative and inconsiderate boss.

Perhaps it was something specific she said, or the way she said it, that upset you to the point where when you were at home in the evening, you felt the urge to eat comfort food, thoughts of your favorites arising unbidden from the depths of your primitive brain.

We all have the need to feel appreciated for our efforts. Napoleon famously said that men are led by baubles, meaning that they would risk their lives for shiny medals. His observation was entirely correct; appreciation is that important to us.

So it is quite possible that your unappreciative boss's comment was your emotional trigger, and that the unmet need this indicates is your need for appreciation.

It may, however, be that the cause of your emotional distress is something deeper.

It is human nature to look for a reason when we feel upset, an explanation for why we feel distress. We look in our environment, and as soon as we discover a potential cause latch upon it as the reason we are unhappy.

For example, we may fly off the handle at a remark from our spouse. We then say that the trigger for our losing our cool is our spouse who fails to show us the proper respect, or is otherwise contrary.

Often the reason that we are upset in any given situation is not the apparent cause but rather a deeper malaise of which we are unaware. The late Dr. Wayne Dyer used to ask, "What do you get when you squeeze an orange?"

Well, you always get orange juice because that's what's inside it.

By this he meant to remind us that, if we are expressing, in our example, anger, it means that anger was inside of us.

The remark by our spouse may have been what "squeezed" us, but our spouse wasn't necessarily the source of the anger any more than the person squeezing the orange is the source of the juice.

That's why you have to look deeper for the cause of your emotional distress rather than accepting what appears obvious at first blush.

Once you have determined the emotional trigger which gave rise to your primitive brain urging you to overeat, you must next look at what activities you are drawn to as soothing alternatives to food.

In our example of our boss's lack of appreciation for our efforts, while it is a legitimate need for humans to be appreciated, we can look at what soothing activities we are drawn to for an indication of what we lack.

If we are drawn to social alternatives to food — perhaps we call a friend, who listens to us and reassures us that we are important and valuable and are to be appreciated for the sincere efforts we make to do our work well — then it's likely true that our unmet emotional need is for appreciation.

However, if we instead are drawn to, for example, creativity as a soothing alternative to food we may be lacking the human need for control or creative expression.

It could be that the nature of our work — perhaps it is repetitive, tedious, stultifying or otherwise frustrating to us — filled us with negative emotions which our boss merely released with her unappreciative comment.

We may have an unmet need, not for appreciation — although certainly appreciation is always nice — but rather for control of our work process, or an unmet need for creativity.

It is important to drill down to determine exactly what unmet emotional need is filling our "orange" with negative emotion.

This takes some doing. It takes patience, and the ability to explore without judgment, or rather while reserving judgment, both the stresses in our environment and the soothing activities to which we are drawn.

Fortunately, the unmet needs that are most significant in our lives will be the ones that surface most often.

We don't have to wonder what it is that we most lack, as it will become readily apparent if we simply pay attention.

We have not one, but many examples of emotional triggers which we can consider — our primitive brain is relentless at urging us to engage in emotional eating when it perceives emotional discord.

If we explore our choices each time we have food cravings or otherwise experience the urge to engage in emotional eating, we will soon have sufficient data to determine our most significant unmet needs.

For example, if we continue to be drawn to creativity as a soothing food alternative regardless of the emotional trigger involved, then we could safely assume that this was the unmet need which filled us with negative emotions.

If it only applied to triggers arising from our workplace, then we would be able to define it further and be able to state with some confidence that it was a problem of our work giving rise to an unmet need, specifically that for control or creative expression.

It is likely that there is more than one unmet need in your life. There may be one predominant unmet need which will arise time and time again, but you will almost certainly notice others.

The wonderful thing about the primitive brain, and the reason it is such a tremendous ally in your search to uncover the unmet needs in your life, is that is indefatigable in its quest to ensure that its survival drives are heeded.

You do not *need* to heed them, and indeed you have learned the EEESY™ way to gain the upper hand with your primitive brain.

But its voice will never go away. At the first sign of distress, it will be there to remind you that you can instantly soothe yourself by consuming food and jettisoning your eating plan.

Even as you meet your most important needs, other, less important needs will make their presence known. Since you are human and imperfect, there will be no end to this. But your life will improve with each need you determine and meet.

Your emotional eating will be a thing of the past, but you will still be relying on it to be able to detect what's missing in your life and to remind you to take proactive steps to correct the deficit.

You can do this in an atmosphere of complete safety. There is no external threat to your well-being involved.

Most other reminders that you require self-improvement come from external sources and arrive with negative consequences.

But for you, the urgings of your primitive brain to engage in emotional eating, has no consequence at all — apart from the need for you to use EEESY™ and engage in soothing alternatives to eating, many of which have some benefit to us — and you are thus able to improve ourselves proactively, and meet your needs, without risk or penalty.

You are in complete control and can proceed at your own pace, and in a manner with which you are comfortable.

Contrast this safe proactive approach to self-improvement, meeting the needs in your life which are lacking and which cause you emotional pain, with the reactive approach to personal change which is the more common experience.

Persons in recovery will often attribute their desire for change to their "hitting bottom;" that the utter destruction they experienced was their motivation for seeking help.

They are often grateful for whatever dramatic negative consequence finally drove them to go to Alcoholics Anonymous or enter a recovery program.

Wouldn't it be so much better to proactively address the problems at the root of our emotional distress?

Wouldn't it be preferable to seek self-improvement before we suffered severe consequences?

And wouldn't it be better still, if instead of trying to avoid hitting bottom we were reaching for the stars?

By employing your primitive brain as an ally to determine your unmet needs, you will be able to uncover them one at a time, and as you meet them, you will progressively become a happier and more fulfilled human being.

This process is the diametric opposite of the cycle of emotional eating; it is the diametric opposite of the cycle of any addiction.

It is a virtuous cycle, not a vicious one, and it can lead you to a fuller, richer, more joyful life.

So take the time you need to determine your needs.

Each time you feel the stirrings of your primitive brain urging you to eat contrary to your eating plan use EEESY™ and then look for the emotional trigger that engaged your primitive brain's survival drives, and explore the food alternatives to which you are drawn to soothe yourself, and the choices that you made.

Drill down.

Don't be satisfied with the most obvious answer but look for deeper needs that may be being masked, which you can find if you continue to look at your emotional triggers and the choices you make to address them each time your primitive brain urges you to engage in emotional eating.

Be as relentless in digging out your deepest needs as your primitive brain is in reminding you that something you need is missing in your life.

Sometimes an Intervention is Necessary

This is an area where it is particularly helpful to have someone you can lean on. Choose someone who is close to you at the beginning of your process, at the moment you know that you are going to change your lifestyle, and notify him or her. Think of this person as your friendship helpline. Tell them you may be calling them at random times and confirm that this person's life can accommodate potentially coming over at 2am to help you (this is taking into consideration that your friend may have an addiction of their own, a newborn, etc.). That way, if you ever feel you are not strong enough to handle a self-intervention on your own, you will have someone you can call.

Doubt

Sometimes it may feel like no matter what you do, nothing is working. What you may not realize is that by simply making attempts to change your lifestyle, you have already begun to change your mindset. There are small things that may need to be changed in regards to your road to recovery; perhaps you don't like going to workout classes and would prefer to have one-on-one sessions with a friend, or maybe you need to distance yourself from familiar people and instead talk with a group that can relate to your issues. Whatever those changes may be, they are still aides that are helping you to heal yourself and so are doing you some good even if they feel useless. Remember that healing doesn't always feel good because in order to heal, you must confront negative experiences and emotions. In order to give yourself permission to be happy and satisfied with yourself, you must first realize that you have not given yourself that luxury before and you must come to terms with why that is.

Sometimes doubt is used as a shield from the things we fear. If you find yourself doubting that recovery is possible, ask yourself why. Do you fear failing or change? Create a journal listing your doubts and fears; expand on them and then speak to a licensed medial professional regarding what you wrote. They may be able to alleviate some of your fears and navigate you through the recovery process. It may be also helpful to write yourself a note in the journal, detailing your hopes for the future. Similar to the mantra repeated in the mirror, write down what you like about yourself and that you love yourself. Rereading this message will help to tear down any doubts that are based in self-loathing. Remember, you have incredible value and can absolutely overcome BED.

Whenever you are feeling moments of doubt, again, talk to someone about it. It may also be highly useful to speak to a professional who can help you sort through the feelings of doubt and the emotional burden that comes with it, regardless of writing journal entries. But the most important thing to remember is this: no matter how you are feeling about the path you are on, do not give up. Your entire future depends on whether or not you give up binge eating, and while it may be the hardest struggle of your life, you will eventually thank yourself for it. Additionally, no one ever healed himself or herself in one day. It can take a long time to recover from binge eating, emotionally, physically, and mentally, so you must give yourself permission to take your time. Do what is best for you and eventually, things will start to get better.

Relapsing

This is going to happen; there is no denying it. If breaking a food addiction were easy than many people would have gotten rid of theirs by now. The thing is, it's not easy, you will most likely make a mistake, and that's ok.

So when the time comes that you do make a mistake, what do you do about it? First, create distance between yourself and the food you are binging on. Get out of the house and take a walk, something to help you take your mind off of food. When you concentrate on something else, your need to think obsessively about food will naturally decline because the brain can only concentrate on so much at once. So after you have gotten out of the house or sat down in the living room and started furiously working on a crossword, think about what led you to binge. Were you upset about something? Did you mistake your hunger for thirst and then find yourself unable to stop? Identify the reasons for slipping up so that you can have a plan to confront those same situations in the future.

It may also be helpful to utilize your friendship helpline at this time. If you feel like you can't stop eating or want to return to the kitchen, don't be afraid to get on the phone and ask for help. No one expects you to be able to heal yourself completely on your own and that is an unfair burden to put on yourself. Allow yourself to accept help and to talk to someone about your feelings, then pick yourself up and start over.

Preventing a Relapse

Relapsing will happen on the road to healing and is a perfectly normal part of the process, which is part of the reason why it is so important to not beat yourself up when a relapse occurs. Knowing this, it is imperative that you create a plan in order to foresee a potential relapse and know what to do when you feel one coming on.

- *You find yourself obsessing over food, your diet, or weight.*

- *You begin substituting eating for other obsessive behaviors as a way to exercise control.*

- *You feel trapped by your stress and unable to release it in a healthy manner.*

- *You obsess over your body using a mirror or weight scale.*

- *You plan your day around food.*

- *Meals are followed by crushing guilt or shame.*

If you feel any of these items are holding true to your feelings, you may indeed be at risk for a relapse. If you do find that this is the case, you must immediately talk to someone about it. The fact that you are struggling with the idea of overeating indicates that you know you are in danger, and also indicates that you probably need some help dealing with the issues at hand, which there is no shame in. So if you do feel a relapse coming on, first get on the phone with a friend, parent, sibling, other relative, or a professional, just as long as you can speak about your concerns with someone you trust immediately.

After you have spoken with someone, pay attention to what your body needs. Are you really hungry? If you are, then don't be afraid to give yourself some nutrients as long as you are mindful of how much you are eating. Again, eat slowly and purposefully, without shaming yourself. Cutting yourself off from food as a solution to binge eating may only result in other potential eating disorders and may even contribute to more binging in the future because you are denying your body fuel. So monitor how much you are eating in order to satiate your hunger but avoid binging. If it helps, go ahead and count the calories that you need as long as it does not become obsessive; again, we want to avoid addictive behavior. Once more, do not judge yourself, but be sure to treat yourself with compassion.

Lastly, one of the best ways to prevent a relapse is to create a safety net at the beginning of your recovery process and realize your limitations. Create a team to help you on your way back to health, including the person you have selected for your friendship helpline and your therapist. Other trusted individuals to add to your team could be a parent, sibling, mentor, or someone from a support group who can act as a kind of sponsor. Choose people you trust; rely on this team and confide in them if you fear you are beginning to relapse. If they vocalize concern for your well-being, pay attention and heed their advice, even if you think you are in a healthy place. Remember that you have selected them for their aid and support; trust that they want what's in your best interest. Recovery from BED is an ongoing process that requires continuous support and self-reflection. With help from your team, you have a better chance of preventing relapses and the added benefit of not having to go through this ordeal alone.

Juggling Addiction

In some cases, those who suffer from binge eating are juggling multiple addictions or disorders that can leave them feeling crippled. Common among these is depression, personality disorders, and anxiety, but can also include smoking, drinking, gambling, or other addictions. Many binge eaters also force themselves to partake in strenuous diets and exhausting exercise routines that further contribute to binge eating.

According to addiction researcher and journalist Stanton Peele at *Psychology Today*, binge eating—as well as sex—are strangely not included in the DSM-5 despite there being millions of cases in which people have become addicted to food and sexual activities. The reason for the exclusion of these two items is that, unlike drugs or gambling, they are considered to be "universal appetites," or natural parts of life. However, this could also be argued of alcohol. Many people partake in alcoholic substances, but it is the amount and frequency in addition to the underlying reason why someone drinks that categorizes an addiction to alcohol. While sex addiction has been excluded from the DSM-5 completely, BED has been placed in an isolated category outside of addiction.

Because one of the major suggestions for fighting the hunger, guilt, and deprivation that comes with conquering binge eating is to find distractions or other activities in which to engage rather than consuming large amounts of calories, there is the possibility of developing additional addictions or addictions as substitutes for overeating. For example, instead of binge eating, a person may find themselves spending hours each day in casinos pouring their money into slot machines, or taking up smoking, or hoarding in order to avoid confronting their true emotions, instead attempting to fill the void that was once filled by overeating with a different addiction.

If you fall into this category, particularly if you suffer from substance abuse disorder, you must consult a medical professional in order to make sure that your plan for recovery does not compromise your health. Some things to avoid may be strenuous exercise that will quickly exhaust your lungs or put too much stress on your organs. Additionally, you will have to pay special attention that you do not substitute one addiction for another. For example, if you stop binging but start smoking a pack of cigarettes every day, then your health will merely decline in a different way. Additionally, taking up a new addiction will only aid the addictive traits that you are trying to dissipate. It is highly advised that you seek professional medical help in order to approach your recovery in a health-conscious way.

Binging and Purging

Binging and purging, also known as bulimia, is a condition in which a person overeats in the same way as a person with BED, but proceeds to rid the body of the food consumed through forced regurgitation.

The second behavior characteristic of those struggling with bulimia is normally executed in one of two ways: self-induced regurgitation or the use of laxatives. The majority (between 70% and 80%) of those with bulimia prefer the self-induced vomiting method. The side effects associated with the self-induced purging strategy include dental corrosion, potassium deficiency, bursting blood vessels in the eyes, abrasions in the esophagus, and deadly interruptions in heart rhythm.

Approximately 30% of those with bulimia resort to using laxatives, especially the type that specifically affect bowel movements. Breaking free from a binging and purging cycle that involves laxatives can be tricky due to the side effects that go along with the body's adjustment to laxatives. When the body becomes used to laxatives, ceasing use could cause stomach pain, bloating, and constipation. Just like self-induced vomiting, laxatives can lead to potassium deficiency that causes severe fatigue and lack of energy in addition to dehydration, which is another cause of constipation. In severe cases of weaning the body off laxatives, the bowel can become completely unresponsive. Since laxatives are not meant for regular use in any dosage, the safest way to overcome an addiction to them is to cease use completely "cold turkey." Depending on the severity of the laxative addiction, some minor side effects are to be expected but your digestive system and your bowels should return to normal working order within approximately 10 days. If the side effects persist beyond 10 days, you should consult your primary care physician immediately.

Food Blackouts

In the case of some people struggling with BED, "food blackouts" can occur in which individuals are unable to recall an episode or episodes of binge eating. This lasts until the individual enters the kitchen and discovers stacks of dirty dishes and piles of empty food packages lying around and conclude that they have partaken in a binge the night before. These blackouts are often due to an individual's attempts to avoid overeating while battling cravings throughout the day for foods that are high in calories and low in nutritional content. When trying to ignore cravings and adjust to a lower daily calorie intake, it is not uncommon to give into temptation by the end of the day and gorge yourself, sometimes to the point of blacking out. Those who experience these food blackouts while battling BED are prone to feelings of guilt, shame, hopelessness, and helplessness; however, it is not impossible to defeat this.

The first order of business when faced with the guilt and shame of a food blackout is to understand that the act of binge eating is not something that occurs due to weakness or not enough willpower and that binge eating is an addiction—an illness—that you did not choose to acquire. Food blackouts are partly due to your brain and body being conditioned to binging, so when an episode occurs, you are on a sort of mental autopilot or cruise control without being aware of what you are doing. Therefore, the next step in avoiding food blackouts is to understand that binge eating and any associated negative thoughts and behaviors are abnormal.

The body can heal itself.

The body is one of the smartest machines known to man. If the body is sick, the white blood cells rush in to make it better. If there is a cut or wound, the immune system is strong enough to restore it. The body is designed to know what it's doing to keep you alive and sustain life. However, our minds got off track of what is healthy and what is pure and as a side effect, the body stops operating like the strongest fat burning machine that it is.

Listen, we can battle this until the cows come home, but what I know for sure is that if you put nutrient dense foods in your body, the body will start working in the way that it should and eventually start repairing every cell and every tissue in your body. Just like you are the product of your environment, the environment that you create for your body is important too.

Every month, every molecule in your body is replaced. Think about what that means. Everything is replaced in your body. The skin on your hands is replaced every thirty days and the inside of your stomach every six weeks is made anew. You were a different person last month, than you are this month and the only reason you are the way that you are and the environment is the way that is it for you is because you are not willing to do anything about it to change.

Health starts in the kitchen and it starts with what is in front of your plate. It is time to make a shift in your beliefs of what you think is healthy and what you can do to change your health if it's not.

Since the 1930s and the rave of the fast food industry, people have been starving. An oxymoron to say since one-third of the population is obese and America has been going hungry daily.

The foods that we once had are not the same anymore and researchers now say that the parents are going to outlive their children. How scary is that? When making this convenient seemed to make things easier for the average

America is now causing each household more problems not only in their health but in their finances as well.

Did you know that on an annual basis 652,486 deaths are caused by heart disease and that 533,888 people are dying from cancer? Those numbers seem staggering and shocking because those deaths could have been avoided.

Again, this book is made not to convert you to becoming a vegetarian or going 100% raw, but it's simply to do this—to share a message of hope with the nation and to be able to provide solutions to people who have been searching for them. What we are doing here is helping you see that there are real answers out there and people that are out there every day ready to help you get underway with your own personal transformation.

It is not about how much weight you lose or what healthy habit you are going to instill in yourself, but how strong are you going to become at the end of your journey. Are you going to push yourself forward when you think you can't? It is about developing your inner strength and seeing what you are capable of doing.

Not too long ago I was sitting on the plane heading back home from a long trip and I was sitting next to these two women who were obese and I didn't say anything but I noticed what they were eating. They brought with them two massive bags of potato chips and soda and they told me it was a healthy lunch. Of course it was an overnight flight and I didn't want to get into a conversation with them, but it made me think of how brainwashed people really are. It also made me think about how food has a powerful effect on why people get food addictions in the first place.

Food addiction does not just manifest. It happens over time with certain kinds of food that alter the vibration of the body.

Sugar and caffeine are just a few examples that can potentially trigger addictions and compulsive eating.

This book is not about taking away your favorite foods, but rather give you some powerful tools that you can use daily to empower you to make new choices. The most obvious is this; you need to avoid soda and all those sugary drinks.

Although this transformation is going to be dramatic, it's not going to be done in a dramatic way. It is something that is easy and something anyone can do. Most importantly, it is affordable and convenient to your lifestyle.

People these days are so far from the truth that sometimes when an answer is right in front of them, they reject it. Frequently without realizing it people are depositing into their bodies toxins and waste that they are not even aware of how a healthy body should feel like. If you are not detoxifying the liver, you cannot process or absorb nutrients for your body.

The best way to detox is to use a method that supports the liver function while it removes impurities, but it also provides you with a clinically proven blend of vitamins and minerals as well as antioxidant phytonutrients that enhances your immunity overall.

Here is what I supplement with: *http://j.mp/vhealthy*

Cleansing begins with juicing. The best juicer I can recommend for you to use is the *Omega 8006*. Not only does it juice wheatgrass, but all of your favorite vegetables like kale, spinach, dandelions and all sorts of abundant fruit.

Exercise at least three times a week for about ten minutes and have alkaline foods in the morning to boost your energy throughout the day.

When we change the way we eat and begin the process of transforming our body, we can also start the process of healing ourselves on an emotional level and how the world sees us. I believe that there is a global shift happening on the planet where people are starting to wake up and become more aware of who they are. People are starting to realize that they are more than just their physical self.

This leads me to my next statement which is; when you change the energy of how you show up in the world, you will bend the Universe at will. All healing of any kind, whether it is from emotional scarring, compulsive eating or addictions, all starts on a spiritual level, not the physical. Healing starts with an intention and not from a head-space.

Complementary Therapies

Acupuncture

Acupuncture is an ancient form of traditional Chinese medicine in which fine needles are inserted into key points of the body, located along what are known as energy or meridian lines. It is not a stand-alone therapy for eating disorder treatment but is used as an adjunct to other psychological and or medical approaches.

The philosophy behind this treatment is that the manipulation of fine needles within various sites (which supposedly relate to specific organs in the body) will rebalance the body's energy flow. It is a holistic approach that can increase a client's sense of well-being on a physical and emotional level. The client's improved welfare is then believed to increase their receptiveness to formal treatments.

Acceptance and commitment therapy (ACT)

ACT is a derivative of cognitive behavioural therapy (CBT) that incorporates mindfulness. In ACT, the client is taught how to acquire a healthier attitude toward their body image and eating behaviours. By teaching mindfulness, in which clients become increasingly aware of their own thoughts and feelings, they become adept at early identification of destructive patterns and can choose not to react.

This level of insightfulness makes it easier for them to intercept and challenge the ingrained negative thought patterns that automatically lead to impulsive behaviours, such as bingeing and purging. By being aware of the triggers in their environment that activate negative body image beliefs and feelings, an individual can learn to apply a more positive and flexible attitude and can break destructive cycles of behaviour.

Hypnotherapy

Hypnotherapy is a very powerful tool for helping people to overcome eating disorders. By inducing a form of locked attention, a hypnotherapist can help a sufferer to focus on their problem in a heightened state of concentration. Hypnosis is an induced state of trance that artificially activates the brain's REM (rapid eye movement) state. While in this highly focused state, the hypnotherapist uses guided imagery to help induce a state of relaxation. The client is then better able to use the right hemisphere of the brain, which is creative, adept at problem-solving and capable of new learning.

Contrary to popular belief, hypnosis does not involve taking over someone else's mind. Hypnosis facilitates the individual's own ability to lock attention onto an idea and deal with it in a creative manner. In this way, new constructive forms of behaviour can be explored in a safe and non-threatening fashion. It is easy to visualize the potential of this form of treatment for someone who has been locked in negative eating habits like bingeing or laxative misuse.

Kinesiology

This is a form of energy work that seeks to rebalance the body's bio-energetic field to enable the body to heal. By using a combination of nutrition, energy reflexes, emotional techniques and massage, blockages in the energy flow are believed to be removed and the system is rebalanced. This holistic approach claims to be able to help discover the root cause of the client's problem, be it emotional, physical or chemical. This approach is used in conjunction with other treatments to address the eating disorder.

Massage

Clients with eating disorders often perceive their body as the enemy. Massage enables a client to experience their physical being in a pleasant and relaxing way, which helps to foster a more positive and healthy body image. The relaxation and releasing of tension in the body that accompanies massage also helps to reduce stress levels.

Remedial massage involves the masseur manipulating the client's body in a methodical, systematic manner, which serves to increase their dopamine and serotonin levels. Dopamine and serotonin play key roles in reward-motivated behaviour by contributing to feelings of happiness and well-being, which in turn help to alleviate depression.

Deep abdominal massage focuses on the tissue in this region, enabling tension to be released from both the reproductive and digestive systems. People suffering from bulimia in particular can find considerable relief in this form of massage as it can help to activate a sluggish digestive system.

Indian head massage is an ancient practice that is particularly effective in reducing stress and depression as well as decreasing insomnia in sufferers of eating disorders. Since it does not involve the removal of clothing or the need for a special massage table, it can be delivered in any environment and may be useful for sufferers who are uncomfortable about removing their clothes.

Meditation

Meditation can take many different formats, but all types help to promote self-acceptance and increase bodily awareness. Meditation provides the client with a means of self-soothing so that they can reduce their agitation by focusing on their breathing or repeating a mantra.

For clients with eating disorders, this adjunct to other therapies can help sufferers to reconnect with hunger signals and signals of satiety, with which they have lost touch. It is believed that by learning to transform their mental attitudes they will be able to release their own innate powers for self-healing.

By increasing self-awareness, meditation enables the sufferer to arrest destructive eating patterns that have become habitual. Learning how to meditate is a hugely useful practice for people who have addictions and is therefore particularly helpful for those suffering from binge eating disorder.

Neurolinguistic programming (NLP)

Neurolinguistic programming is a treatment that seeks to change the language we use in our mind. By reprogramming our minds, we are able to impose new positive patterns of thought, which in turn enable us to change our behaviour and produce more constructive results.

This approach uses techniques such as hypnosis and positive affirmation to reprogramme the unconscious mind, disrupting deeply established bad habits and internalizing new beneficial habits.

A compulsive habit, such as self-induced vomiting after bingeing, is perpetuated as a consequence of the sufferer's self-perception. NLP reprogrammes the mind and attitude of the sufferer so that they can value themself differently and employ more constructive behaviours. Many people suffering from eating disorders find NLP to be very empowering, not only in helping them to conquer their eating disorder but also in their lives generally.

Reflexology

Reflexology is one of the most popular forms of bodywork –
therapies and techniques in complementary medicine that
involve touching or manipulating the body. Although there is no
scientific proof to support this practice, there is a great wealth of
anecdotal evidence that it promotes deep relaxation.

A reflexologist will apply pressure to various points on the ears,
hands or feet, which allegedly represent other parts of the body.
For example, the foot is divided up into various zones, each zone
corresponding to the digestive system, heart or other organs. By
applying a specific sequence of pressure to each zone, the aim is
to rebalance the client's body.

Reiki

Reiki is another form of energy work, but it is different from
other energy-based modalities in that it is applied with no
specific intent, meaning the energy is non-directed. Reiki was
used during the Gulf War as a way of increasing the sense of
well-being of those in the military. It is a hands-on therapy that
is quick and easy to apply.

By means of therapeutic touch, administered by the practitioner
on the clothed body of the client, the body's energetic field is
rebalanced; this promotes, calmness, clarity, relaxation and
stress relief.

When used in conjunction with other forms of therapy, the soothing practice of reiki can help to empower sufferers of eating disorders to approach their recovery with greater mental, physical and emotional strength.

Yoga

Yoga refers to a range of physical, mental and spiritual disciplines practised in order to attain peace of mind or to reach a higher state of consciousness or enlightenment.

Yoga practice can be very useful for someone suffering from an eating disorder, since an individual with an eating disorder is so far removed from peace of mind and is certainly not in tune with their true self.

In addition, yoga provides an appropriate form of exercise, particularly suitable for those who compulsively exercise when their body does not possess sufficient calories to meet such strenuous demands. This is often the case for sufferers of anorexia, and gentler forms of yoga can provide a substitute to keep the body flexible and mobile.

Yoga promotes physical and mental self-awareness through physical movement, which helps the client to constructively reconnect with their body. Since sufferers of eating disorders have a jaundiced view of their body image, this can help ground them and achieve a greater degree of self-acceptance.

Furthermore, yoga can enable sufferers of eating disorders to become more consciously aware of pain signals from their body. I know of several over-exercisers who have continued to work out frenetically despite sprains, strains and blisters, seemingly unaware of their body's physical cues. Yoga helps reset this awareness and makes the sufferer less likely to exercise to a point that causes physical damage.

In most of these techniques, the underpinning science is largely irrelevant if the practice achieves a positive outcome. Taking care of oneself and feeling deserving of time and attention is in itself enormously therapeutic and increases self-esteem.

Sufferers of eating disorders often do not feel worthy of such attention, and the act of receiving and accepting care in this way is particularly beneficial in helping them to change their harsh attitudes towards themselves.

Conclusion

There are different causes of overeating, including psychological, emotional, chemical, and physiological. There is no good reason to eat until you are uncomfortable. While nearly everyone overeats once in a while, overeating regularly and feeling unable to stop even when you are full can be a problem.

Left unchecked, overeating habits can often result in major health issues. It is important to make a commitment to control your eating habit. Gain control of your urges to overeat and stop this bad behavior before it ruins your health and well-being. Use these simple steps to help you stop overeating once and for all.

As you embark on the journey to overcome overeating, it is important to point out that the journey will not be easy. You will have moments when you relapse, overeat, and feel bad about yourself and even want to binge even the more. However, you need to pick yourself up, learn from your mistakes, and implement effective guidelines that will help you stay on track. You will also have moments when you think that it is too hard and you just want to give up. During such times, remember how far you have come and get the motivation to move on by looking at all the benefits you start to benefit. It is also important that you get some form of support, as it is very hard to overcome any addiction without any help. Your family and friends, as well as online forums, can be a source of great support.